YogaBellies. For Pregnancy

Your Yoga, Nutrition and Wellness Bible for Pregnancy

By

Cheryl MacDonald

Foreword by Maha al Musa

Legal Notes

Copyright © 2015

All rights reserved. No part of this book may be reproduced, stored in a retrieval system, or transmitted in any form or by any means, electronic, mechanical, photocopying, recording, scanning, or otherwise, without the prior written permission of the publisher.

Disclaimer

All the material contained in this book is provided for educational and informational purposes only. No responsibility can be taken for any results or outcomes resulting from the use of this material.

While every attempt has been made to provide information that is both accurate and effective, the author does not assume any responsibility for the accuracy or use/misuse of this information.

ISBN- 13: 978-1517365837
ISBN- 10: 151736583X
BISAC: Health & Fitness / Pregnancy & Childbirth

YogaBellies for Pregnancy

Your Yoga, Nutrition and Wellness Bible for Pregnancy

By Cheryl MacDonald

Foreword by Maha al Musa

If you'd like to download a free YogaBellies for Pregnancy video routine, just
pop your email address in here

Contents

Dedication 7

Foreword by Maha al Musa 8

YogaBellies, Community and Pregnancy 9

Pregnancy Care the YogaBellies Way 12

Ayurveda in Pregnancy 18

Pregnancy Nutrition for Mum and Baby 26

    The Foods You Should Be Loving During Pregnancy 26

    Say 'Bye-Bye' to these Foods During Pregnancy! 28

    Always Make a Shopping List 30

Yoga and Exercise in Pregnancy 32

Yoga and Exercise in Pregnancy 33

    10 Reasons Why You Need to Exercise During Pregnancy 33

    Choosing an Exercise Programme for Pregnancy 35

    Why YogaBellies Is So Much More Than Exercise for Pregnancy 38

    Six Reasons Why Pregnancy Yoga is Even Better in the Water 45

    Preparing to Practice Yoga During Pregnancy 47

    Getting Started with YogaBellies for Pregnancy 54

    Creating your Pregnancy Yoga Space 57

Pranayama (Breathing) for Pregnancy 59

    Top Tips for Pregnancy Pranayama 59

    Beautiful Breathing for Pregnancy 60

    Ujjayi Breathing (oo-Ji-EE) 60

    Nadi Shodana (nah-dee shod-an-a) - Alternate Nostril Breathing .. 61

    Brahamarri (brahm-ar-ee) - Humming Bee Breath 62

YogaBellies for Pregnancy Meditation... Meet your Baby 63

    Why Should I Meditate During Pregnancy? 63

The First Trimester and Getting to Know Your Pregnant Self 66

    What's Happening with Mum and Baby in the First trimester? 67
    Recommended Foods for the First Trimester 69
    Pregnancy Smoothie Power! 69
    Meal Plans for the First Trimester 70
    YogaBellies in the First Trimester 76

The Second Trimester and Crazy Cravings 84
    What's Happening with Mum and Baby in the Second Trimester? ... 85
    Recommended Foods for the Second Trimester 86
    Meal Plans for the Second Trimester 87
    YogaBellies in The Second Trimester 92
    What's Happening with Mum and Baby in the Third Trimester? 96
    Recommended Foods for the Third Trimester 97
    Meal Plans for The Third Trimester 98
    YogaBellies in the Third Trimester 107
    Nutrition in Pregnancy: QUICK REMINDERS 111

The Fourth Trimester and Post-Partum Mama 112
    Ayurveda for Postpartum Mama 113
    Rocking Your Beautiful New Body 117
    Post Natal Yoga: With and Without Baby 120
    Some Signs that You're Not Ready to Practice Yet 124
    Bringing Movement Back into Your Life 125

YogaBellies 129

Post-Natal BAP's Routines 129
    Finding Ways to Fit Your Yoga Practice Around Your Baby 133
    Beyond The Baby Blues 133

Final Thoughts 136

Yoga Glossary 139

References 143
    About the Author 146

Other books by the Author..149
YogaBellies for Pregnancy DVD...152

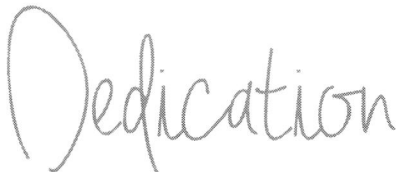

I would like to dedicate this book to all beautiful YogaBellies teachers and YogaBellies mamas, who have inspired me to put pen to paper and continue to inspire me every single day.

I would like to give a special thanks to Jennifer MacDonald and Sophie Keil, who helped me to put this book into a readable format. And of course my two special boys, my husband and my gorgeous son, Caelen.

Foreword by Maha al Musa

Are you ready to be guided by the loving hand and heart of a compassionate and caring woman on your pregnancy and birthing journey? Do you wish to be lovingly held by the beauty of your sister's gifts? If so you have found the right book that will practically and gently open these doorways into your own knowing - Cheryl McDonalds YogaBellies for Pregnancy.

As founder of Bellydance for Birth - mindful movement to awaken birth wisdom - since 1997 - I am passionate about keeping the thread of women's knowledge alive for pregnancy, birth and mothering. The language of the feminine must be available to all women on this rite of passage journey. Cheryl and I are both passionate about sharing with women our insights and wisdoms so they feel supported and comforted with an emphasis on practical movement as well as spiritual guidance.

Within the pages of this book Cheryl generously captures this essence for all pregnant mummas. She beautifully and compassionately guides you through the stages of pregnancy and post-partum care using the principles of Ayurveda and ancient yoga to create a practical, comprehensive and invaluable resource to support you and your babies blossoming.

As Cheryl writes Ayurveda says "we are what we digest" and she has, through her book, given all women a calm and soothing place to digest the experience of pregnancy and birth for optimum physical and psychological attunement. I highly recommend YogaBellies for Pregnancy.

Maha Al Musa Sacred somatic prenatal and birth educator.
Founder of Bellydance for Birth - The Al Musa Method - since 1997
www.mahaalmusa.com

YogaBellies, Community and Pregnancy

Thanks to the mass media circus and horror stories you may have heard from well-meaning friends, pregnancy and birth have become the most dreaded times in a woman's life. When I started YogaBellies, I wanted to found a community to take women away from this negativity. I wanted to encourage women to experience yoga that was so much more than pulling some shapes on a yoga mat. I wanted to support and guide my fellow mothers', using yoga as a foundation for a healthy and happy pregnancy.

I am always keen to dispel outdated stereotypes about having to be super bendy or a bearded hippy, to practice yoga. I set out to provide yoga classes for women, which were accessible to every level of yoga practitioner; were not terrifying and were genuinely more than just acrobatics for skinny hippies.

My love of all things pregnancy, birth and yoga, led me to explore yoga for pregnancy and also, hypnobirthing. These combined therapies and a genuine love of my work, brought YogaBellies into being. Women across the UK and then the globe, began to understand how YogaBellies could provide them with support, comfort, health and wellness during the perinatal period. YogaBellies quickly became a community of women supporting women: Our teachers supporting mothers', and mothers' supporting each other, during this amazing but often daunting time. Today, thousands of women across the world attend YogaBellies for Pregnancy classes and embrace the journey towards motherhood for the glorious time that it is.

Practicing yoga postures, breathing, deep relaxation and a natural lifestyle, are the perfect way to enjoy a healthy pregnancy and a positive birth. I love that pregnant women are now embracing natural and holistic ways to stay fit and well throughout the gestation period. Returning to traditional, wholesome and drug free self-care allows pregnancy and birth, to progress as nature intended. It also helps us to promote a faster and safer birth for mum and baby.

Pregnancy and childbirth can of course be hard work, but it is without a doubt, the most amazing and empowering experience that you are ever likely to have. It's worth every single minute of effort. We can't account for special circumstances arising during pregnancy or birth, we can only look after ourselves and our baby in the best way possible. Hopefully this book will provide you with an easy to follow guide to eating a healthy diet; getting started with a pregnancy yoga practice and easing back into movement, in the immediate post-natal period.

Sending you love, light and multiple blessings on this special journey towards motherhood.

Namaste

Cheryl MacDonald

xxx

Cheryl MacDonald is the founder of YogaBellies, creator of the Birth ROCKS Method and author of the best-selling book by the same name. She founded the Birth ROCKS Academy (affectionately known as BRA) She has trained YogaBellies teachers across the world and has been working with birthing women for over ten years. Cheryl is originally from Glasgow and is mum to one lovely six-year-old boy. She currently lives with her two boys in sunny Singapore, and nips across to Bali where she runs yoga retreats for women.

Pregnancy Care, the YogaBellies Way

Pregnancy Care, the YogaBellies Way

Your Guide to This Guide

In writing this book, I have put together a collection of many of the things that helped me during pregnancy and that I have used to support other women. If you've never really thought about looking after yourself or about what you eat before, or even if you are a clean eating, yoga toting vegan, now is the time to get serious about practical pregnancy self-care and nutrition. You are now literally growing your baby from what you put in and do to your body. A baby built from Diet Coke, Big Mac's and sofa lunging, won't be as healthy or well as a baby built from fresh produce and safe movement. Every good thing you do for you; you do for baby too.

This guide covers three key areas, which can offer so much support and nourishment for you and your baby across the four trimesters: Yoga, Nutrition and a little dash of Ayurveda. This book will take you through an introduction to each of these concepts as applied to pregnancy, why they are important and how they can apply to you in your pregnancy.

The book is then split into four trimesters, offering advice; meals plans; yoga practice advice and sequences best suited to that stage of pregnancy. Please remember that no two pregnancies are the same and that everyone feels and looks differently, at every stage. Also just because you suddenly pop into the second trimester, it doesn't mean that things which were comforting or useful in the first trimester, will no longer work for you. Listen to your body and be guided by what feels right. These chapters are meant as general rule, and not the law.

I've provided some 'beginners' insight into Ayurveda, as it relates to pregnancy. We have so much to learn from this awesome and ancient science that can apply to pregnant life today. Our diet plans and guide to nutrition are not based on an Ayurvedic diet plan, but I have explained some of the relevant principles. An Ayurvedic approach to eating and lifestyle are complimentary to your yoga practice and an overall sense of wellbeing, for mother and baby.

All of the yoga routines in this guide, are suitable throughout pregnancy. If it feels okay for you and baby, then the yoga routines in this book will be safe at all times during pregnancy. Please be sure to check with your midwife, physio or GP before beginning any physical exercise in pregnancy.

Welcome to Pregnancy!?

Real life pregnancy can come as a bit of a shock, even if your pregnancy has been planned or if you've been trying for a long time. You may be reading this and thinking, there is NO WAY I can practice yoga and all I can stomach to eat, is chips. I'm sick. I'm tired and I'm swollen up like a balloon. And that's okay too. ☺

I know that having wanted a baby for years and having worked with women having beautiful pregnancies and births, I was quite taken aback by the reality of pregnancy. I had envisioned myself floating around in white yoga clothing (yeah right,) cradling my growing bump, looking serene and bonding with my baby in utero, as I had often talked to other mums about. I did not realize that's spend most of my days feeling or being sick!

I suffered from hyperemesis gravidarium (or extreme pregnancy nausea and vomiting) from around six weeks' gestation, which lasted until I was almost eight months pregnant. So the floaty white outfits were a no-go straight away!

Sick of feeling sick?

The constant sickness was a real shocker for me: What happened to my perfect pregnancy and birth?? I knew how to take care of myself before conception and during pregnancy. I had mentored so many other mums through peaceful pregnancies and beautiful births, so what had happened to my vision of pregnancy perfection? But like everything in life, pregnancy and birth are often not as we planned, even if we do 'know it all.'

The sickness really took its toll and the yoga I imagined I would practice every day, which often consisted of me just lying on my yoga mat having a hormonal sob. Being a yoga teacher and at the time, having a six day a week Ashtanga practice, this was a major change for me. I had always told mums 'pregnancy is not an illness' and here I was, vomiting and unable to attend my place of work on a regular basis.

Finding out what soothes your soul

As the weeks passed, the nausea didn't really get much better. But I continued my yoga practice, gently building up my strength again, practising slow, deep ujjayi breathing and easing slowly out of my downward dog.

I started to manage the nausea and vomiting a little better as my pregnancy progressed. I looked to natural and holistic remedies that could help me, Ayurveda being one area of great support. Cheesy Wotsits were also of great support during my nauseous times, so it's not all clean living.

As I started to find my own little tips and tricks, and as I was able to do a little more yoga, I started to feel more in control of my pregnancy and of what was happening to my body. I started to see the funny side. My friend said I was the sickest, happiest person she knew. I'm sure there is a compliment in there somewhere. Yoga helped to make me stronger, physically and mentally, and to cope with the demands that pregnancy was making on my body and mind.

My pregnancy wasn't the one that I dreamed of, but practising yoga helped me to accept that this was my pregnancy, and I was still going to have my own beautiful little baby to love and care for at the end of it.

Bond with your bump and slow down

I talked constantly to my bump (much to the amusement of work colleagues), singing songs and stroking my belly. I loved feeling my little man moving around, feeling him grow stronger and bigger. Meditation and travelling within to chat with my little man, became such an important aspect of my yoga practice during my pregnancy, as much of the time I couldn't manage any physical practice. I've provided my bonding meditation in this guide too, which was a great comfort to me.

I learned to listen to my body. I accepted that my body no longer wanted to practice dynamic yoga every morning. I swapped my vigorous yoga sessions for a few gentle, aware postures which felt good for me and my baby. I gave into the early evening naps that my body so craved when I came home from work. I ate healthily (when the food would stay put) and changed to a liquid vitamin supplement with folic acid that my stomach could tolerate, instead of the horrible bulky tablets.

And all the time aware of my little man growing in my ever expanding belly. I already loved him so much and couldn't wait to meet him.

Love the pregnant life

What I'm trying to say, is that pregnancy is not always perfect. My sickness was reassurance that my baby boy was taking hold and growing strong.

Acceptance was the key for me and this is what I try to teach to mums who come to my classes during pregnancy today. It could be nausea; it could be accepting that you can't run marathons any more. It could be that you have to slow down and that really, you don't want to be in a blaring nightclub at 5am anymore. Every woman has an aspect of pregnancy that wasn't what they expected or that they have to work at accepting.

Surrender to Parenthood

We need to allow ourselves to surrender to mumhood. Women today are expected to achieve all manner of amazing feats while pregnant: keep working 8am-8pm, go to aerobics, prepare the dinner and look after other kids... the list is endless. In years gone by, women didn't work and their sole responsibility was to have and look after babies, mostly with the help of their mother and grandmother too. Today's early motherhood, is generally very different from this, in the Western World.

The thing that makes us strong, the thing that makes us mums, is our ability to sacrifice what we want, for what is best for our child. The word surrender has connotations of giving up or weakness. Surrendering to pregnancy doesn't mean you are weak: it means you are a strong and loving mum listening to what her body and baby need. Give yourself what you need during pregnancy, be that sleep, some time off work or cheesy Wotsits. And please, please forgive yourself if you don't have that perfect, blissful pregnancy that we see on TV adverts.

Even though I wanted a baby more than anything, I didn't want to be sick every day. By accepting my pregnancy, I found joy in my new pregnant life and yoga practice. I went on to have an amazing five hours long, drug free birth and I will never forget the first moment I looked my little man in the eyes. So no matter how swollen your ankles or how creaky your pelvis becomes, I guarantee you that it's worth every minute.

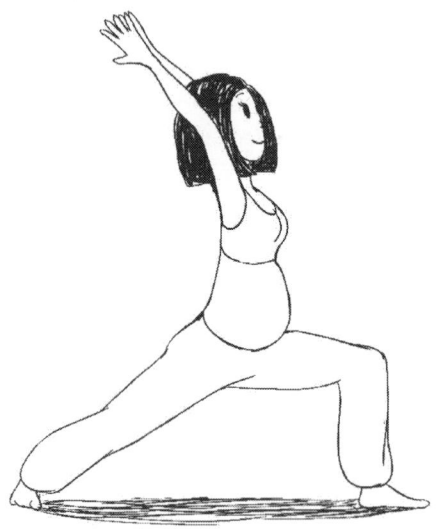

Ayurveda in Pregnancy

Ayurveda in Pregnancy

What is Ayurveda and Why is it Important in Pregnancy?

The word 'Ayurveda' means 'Knowledge of Life' in Sanskrit and is a system of holistic medicine which originated in India around 6,000 years ago. Monks created Ayurveda to improve their physical wellbeing, to allow them to meditate more effectively, which is also the reason that the practice of yoga asana (postures) were introduced. Ayurveda's basic principles can apply to **everybody,** so don't stress if you're not a monk, or have never even heard of it. I'm going to introduce you to some key concepts that will help you have a healthy pregnancy.

According to Ayurveda, everything consists of just five elements: earth, water, fire, air, and space (including us.) Every person has an entirely unique combination of these elements known as their 'Dosha,' loosely translated as body type.

The Doshas:

Vata:

A predominantly Vata constitution will have physical and mental qualities that reflect the elemental qualities of Space and Air. Vata types are often quick thinking, thin, and fast moving.

Pitta:

A Pitta type will have qualities of Fire and Water, such as a fiery personality and oily skin.

Kappa:

A Kappa type will typically have a solid bodily frame and calm temperament, reflecting the underlying elements of Earth and Water.

Everyone consists of varying amounts of each Dosha, with one or two being more prevalent. The Dosha we are more focused on during pregnancy is Vata Dosha, as it is thought to be high in pregnant women and must therefore, be balanced.

During pregnancy, we are not so focused on our just own personal body type (or Dosha,) as there's someone else residing in our body also. We can't be just focused on what our body needs. This guide does not explore the Doshas (that's a huge topic in itself,) but simply draws of the general Ayurvedic guidelines for pregnant women.

Sharing Your Energy

During pregnancy, a downward-moving energy called *apana vata* supports baby's development. If you are looking after yourself and feel balanced and well, then there will be enough *apana vata* for you and baby.

If you've been continuing at your pre-pregnancy pace, eating poorly and have become run down, the upward-moving *vata* – called *prana vata* – has to step in and is redirected downward to support the needs of your baby.

Without prana (energy,) which allows you to embrace and revel in pregnancy, you can be left feeling tired, run down and even depressed. For a healthy pregnancy, the apana and prana vata, should be in balance and that can be achieved only through healthy living.

Nine Months of Self-Loving

In Ayurvedic terms, a pregnant woman is referred to as the 'Garbhini' in Sanskrit and the very special care of a pregnant woman, is known as 'Garbhini Paricharya.' Ayurveda provides a lot of helpful recommendations for women during pregnancy that are fairly consistent from woman to woman. We've popped together some top tips and basic guidance from this amazing science, to help you plan for a nutritious and healthy pregnancy.

In Ayurveda, it is said that a woman can completely reset her health during the childbearing year. It is of the upmost importance that mum takes proper care of herself and baby during this time. However, if you don't make the necessary adjustments to your life to prepare for the changes that lie ahead by ignoring a proper diet, you can create imbalances, that can take a long time to heal. During pregnancy, everything you taste, see, touch, hear, and smell, should be nourishing you. Your environment and general state of mind can affect baby's growth and development.

We have so many things to do as a new mum. A lack of sleep, breastfeeding demands and the constant care your baby, require a whole lot of energy. It is so important that before, during and after pregnancy that you continually look after your general wellbeing.

When you carry a child for nine months, your body does an awful lot of work, and what the baby needs will be taken, directly from your energy stores. Your health must be your first priority.

The three main areas of concerns around health from an Ayurvedic perspective, are food, sleep and how your energy is used. By balancing these three areas throughout pregnancy by watching what you eat, getting ample rest and using your energy well, you will have a healthy body and mind.

Garbh Sanskar: Ayurvedic Pampering in Pregnancy

We all know how important it is to take care of our bodies during pregnancy, so take the time to allow yourself to be pampered. We are carrying precious babes, making our health even more important.

Looking after out body during pregnancy, creates a clean and happy home for baby. Here are some ideas to make you instantly feel better during pregnancy:

- **Get a mani/pedi:** Nothing makes you feel nicer than pretty fingers and toes. If your pregnancy shape and tent-size clothes are getting you down, dressing up and your hands and feet can make you feel pampered and special. Go to a reputable, clean salon and allow then to massage your hands and feet too.
- **Enjoy a massage:** this is best left until after the fifth month. Generally, massages are considered safe in pregnancy and this is a great way to feel pampered and relaxed. Abhygaya massage with lots of oil is perfect. Ideally

visit an Ayurvedic practitioner, but if this is not practical, rope in your partner or a friend to help.
- **Have a bubble bath:** A 'not too warm' bath in pregnancy is safe and very relaxing. I spent most of my first trimester floating around in the tub, and I found that it helped ease nausea also. Find your favourite scent of bubbles, light some few candles, and slide into a warm, bubbly tub.
- **Try out some Bump Photography:** Embrace your pregnancy and go for a glamorous bump photoshoot. You can do this alone or with a friend or partner. Immediate glam appeal and guaranteed to help you love your pregnant body and to serve as a beautiful reminder of your pregnancy.
- **Read a book:** Read those books that you have wanted to for ages. You won't get the chance when baby arrives, so find the time now to do what you love.

Fresh Is Best

The most important principle of Ayurvedic nutrition is that your food is fresh or 'Sattvic.' Ideally your food is free from chemicals, additives and ideally organic. In Ayurveda we also aim to eat food that is 'in season', and where possible, grown locally. This will mean it's less likely to have been frozen or transported thousands of miles.

Fresh food does not have to mean raw food. In Ayurveda, the best way to consume food, is freshly cooked, especially in pregnancy. This is a fantastic approach to eating for mum and baby, meaning that everything they consume is fresh, free from nasties and full of juicy, living energy (prana.) Ayurveda states that food prepared for a pregnant woman should be warm and moist to encourage good circulation. This will also encourage better milk production once baby is born.

Digestion and Pregnancy

What we eat affects our emotions and can create a predisposition for both psychological and physical disorders. Just as wrong emotion can upset our digestion, so wrong digestion can upset our emotions." Dr. David Frawley, Ayurvedic Healing

Digestion in Ayurveda is considered to be the root of all health. During pregnancy, we often suffer from constipation and heartburn, as well as various other digestive ailments, making it even more important.

In the west it is said that we are what we eat. However, in Ayurveda, it's said that we are what we digest. All of the nourishment and energy we have, as well as our emotional well-being, comes from the food that we eat. This is particularly important in pregnancy because the level of nourishment that baby receives, will depend completely on what you eat and how effectively this is digested.

Keep Those Fires Burning Baby

Agni, (meaning Digestive Fire), is regarded in Ayurveda as THE most important concept for healthy digestion. When your Agni is strong, you can easily digest everything that you eat. If your Agni or digestive fire is low, you won't be able to digest your food and your body will produce toxins. I'm sure you can see why a strong Agni is vital in pregnancy!

Sattvic foods are easily digested and nourish the Dhatus (body tissues) of mum and baby. Ensuring that mama has a strong 'digestive fire' is the first step to good health for mum and baby.

Some more Ayurvedic tips for encouraging a healthy Agni or 'digestive fire' include:
- Always aim to eat in a pleasant environment, take your lunch outside if it's a nice day and enjoy the view.
- Focus on eating slowly and not eating while 'on the go;'
- Avoiding overeating because you are eating for two. Think quality, not quantity.
- Avoid foods that are highly stimulating, for example sugars, caffeine or spicy foods.
- Making lunch the biggest meal, as this is when the Agni is naturally at its highest. This helps avoid constipation also;
- Eat several smaller meals or snacks throughout the day to aid digestion;

- Avoid eating leftovers as much as possible as this food will have become stagnant or 'Tamasic.'
- Try to include a good variety of all six tastes (sweet, sour, astringent, bitter, salty, and pungent) at every meal.
- Waiting several hours between meals to ensure that the previous meal has been digested.

Tastes and Craving

In Ayurveda, special attention is given to mum's cravings during pregnancy. It is said that you should be given anything you want to eat (hoorah!) within reason. Whatever we crave during pregnancy, our body and baby need.

Remember, you are eating for two body types now, so you should not follow a strict diet just for you. It is very important to remember to include a good variety of food groups in your diet during pregnancy. For this reason, you should try not eat simply what you always have eaten and to experiment with some healthy, new options.

Ayurvedic Tips for Morning Sickness

As a sufferer of perpetual morning sickness during pregnancy (you can read more about this later,) I know how awful nausea can be. Here are a few fantastic Ayurvedic tips for curbing the queasiness.

- Snack on dry crackers, toast or cheesy wotsits. Keeping something in your stomach curbs the nausea. Even take them into your yoga class, this always helped me.

- Sip a warm tea made with a pinch ginger powder and some fennel seeds.

- Roast and powder cardamom seeds and nibble throughout the day.

- Always try to sleep in a semi-reclined position, use pillows and props as required.

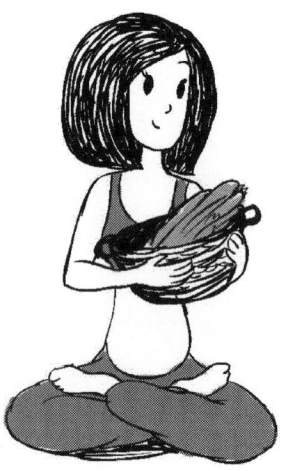

Pregnancy Nutrition for Mum and Baby

Pregnancy Nutrition for Mum and Baby

Just because you are pregnant does not mean you should be 'eating for two,' as in eating two meals where you would have had one. You must consider what you are eating and eat well, this does not equate to doubling your portions and wolfing ten Mars bars every day.

There are probably foods that you know that you should eat, but you wouldn't normally eat or they seem bland and boring. Get some recipe books together and make these food combinations more exciting, but in a positive and healthy way.

You need a lot of good nutrition during pregnancy, but that does not mean you eat everything in sight. Although you should eat more, rules of moderation and variety still always apply.

The Foods You Should Be Loving During Pregnancy

Nutrition is so important for regulating your hormones and your overall wellbeing during pregnancy. When you are pregnant, you still need to fill your own nutritional requirements and also those of your growing baby. I've provided a rundown of some food that's are perfect for a pleasant pregnancy.

Vital Vegetables

Vegetables are a super important part of any pregnant woman's diet, as they provide the body with a lot of carbohydrates. Carbohydrates are the number one nutrient that every pregnant woman needs for hormonal balance, nervous system function and your baby's development.

Carbs are the single most important fuel source for your body. Without them, you will have less energy and will run out of steam quicker. If you generally eat a diet which restricts your carb intake, you may have to up your carb intake to make sure that your body has the energy stores that it needs.

Calcium is another essential vitamin that you need to make sure you are getting lots of during pregnancy. This can be found in abundance in vegetables.

Remember that during pregnancy, you need to eat simple, not complex carbohydrates. Simple carbohydrates are broken down much more efficiently by the body and also ensure you don't put on too much excess weight during pregnancy.

Vegetables like gourd, pumpkin, okra (ladies finger), potatoes and carrots are great. Ayurveda also recommends veggies such as cabbage and gherkins. You should aim to eat vegetables such as green peas, cluster beans, French beans, capsicum, less. Eating too many of these can increases Vata and Pitta. Salads can a great source of vitamins, iron & minerals too, but try not to each too many raw salads, as this could hinder your digestion.

Omega-3 Is Not Optional

Eating fish rich in omega-3, especially DHA, is a great way to assist baby's brain development. Salmon and trout are just two great examples of fish rich in omega-3. There are also pregnancy supplements containing omega-3 which you can purchase over the counter. Eating the right amount of omega-3, will help your baby sleep better and has also been shown to reduce incidence of postpartum depression, after the birth.

Mighty Meat

Meat is a great source of protein during pregnancy. Lean meat is even better as it has a lower amount of fat. Protein is essential in assisting baby's growth over the gestation period and in the worst cases, a protein deficiency can result in birth defects.

Ayurveda recommends Lamb and Chicken as the preferred meats to consume. Always aim to eat high quality, lean meat and stay away from any meat that has a high level of fat. If you are a sausage or bacon lover, try say goodbye for the duration of your pregnancy. Meat is also high in iron. The development of your child's teeth and bones could also be affected in the future, if you don't get sufficient iron.

More Meaty Benefits:
- Keeps your placenta healthy, strong and functioning well;
- Keep's your baby's hormones in check;

- Improves baby's metabolism;
- Encourages breast milk production

Marvellous Milk

Milk is vital to any pregnancy. It contains a huge amount of calcium and is a great source of vitamins A and B. You need to be consuming lots of calcium during pregnancy, as it is essential for your baby's growing heart, muscles, bones and nervous system.

Calcium is not just essential for baby's health. It is essential for you too. Making sure that you have enough calcium in your diet helps to lower blood pressure and can even help you reduce back pain. Calcium is great for easing those pesky pregnancy muscle cramps, and even helps to reduce any discomfort you may experience during birthing. Why wouldn't you want to you drink milk?

This is one of the main reasons why you should never skip breakfast when you are with child. A healthy whole grain cereal with some fresh fruits included, and a glass of freshly squeezed juice, is a great way to start the day if you are pregnant.

Say 'Bye-Bye' to these Foods During Pregnancy!

When you are pregnant, there are quite a few foods you should avoid. I've put together a list of foods that you need to be avoiding for the duration of your pregnancy.

Sometimes when we are pregnant we have crazy cravings, and sometimes we just need to indulge those cravings. Try your best to keep away from the foods listed, but know that if it's only once in a while, it doesn't make you a bad parent... ☺

Ready-Made Rubbish

Anything that is ready to eat, should be completely off limits when you're pregnant. I know that it's often not possible to make everything from scratch, but even try to cook in bulk and freeze some for later. You will be doing nothing but stacking on the calories when you eat pre-packaged food. They tend to be high in salt and extremely unhealthy.

Contrary to popular belief, even 'diet' ready meals and pre-packaged salads, are not a nutritious option. Many of these meals contain a lot of additives and fattening, unhealthy salad dressings too. Although it might be more convenient to buy a salad in the coffee shop at lunch time, try to take the time to make your own salad in advance. It does not take long and it is definitely a lot more nutritious when you know exactly what it contains.

Ice-Cream and Sorbet
Sadly, yet another type of food that you should try to stay away from during pregnancy.

Ice-cream (a personal favourite of mine,) is a particular no-no for women who have gestational diabetes. During pregnancy, the last thing you need is sugary ice-cream. Perhaps look out for a diabetic or sugar free alternative.

Double Check Your Cheese
Soft cheese can contain large amounts of saturated fat which is a pregnant woman's worst enemy. From a health perspective, soft cheeses can contain listeria bacteria and can cause an infection called listeriosis

To avoid any risk, you should not eat any mound-ripened soft cheese such as camembert, brie or soft cheeses made with goats' milk. You should also avoid eating any soft blue-veined cheeses, including Danish blue, Gorgonzola and Roquefort.

Soft cheeses tend to be less acidic than hard cheeses and they also contain more moisture. This means they create an ideal environment for harmful bacteria, such as listeria, to grow.

Terrible Take Away
You've come home from work, you are tired. You just want to phone some take away and get some SLEEP. I get it. If there is one thing you need to try to resist

during pregnancy, its fast food. Everyone knows fast food is a greasy, loaded with fat and additives and generally a cholesterol packed, nasties-filled disaster.

If you want to avoid excessive weight gain and give your baby the best start in life, then keep away from fast food. Eating poorly during pregnancy will mean less stamina, strength and energy for birthing also. And we want to make that as easy as possible, right?

Everything Else to Avoid
- **Avoid** consuming aloe Vera completely, as it can lower your blood sugar levels and even start false contractions.
- Avoid eating too much bread, as well as frozen or canned foods.
- Say no to fermented or stale food.
- Too many cold or aerated drinks should be avoided also.
- Try to avoid any foods with additive colours, spicy and salty foods.

Always Make a Shopping List

When I go shopping, I often forget what I meant to buy and end up buying lots of random things that I didn't need and come home without those I did need. Add baby brain to this and you have the recipe for a shopping disaster! When you are pregnant, you can't afford to buy food that you don't need or should be avoiding. Especially as when we are pregnant we often have the appetite of four!!

If you are determined to avoid unhealthy food and focus on a healthy, nutritious diet, the best thing to do is to make a shopping list. Making a shopping list will ensure that you only buy what you need and that you are not tempted to buy that massive special offer, Dairy Milk.

It can be difficult during pregnancy to remember what food we should be eating and which ones we need to avoid. Team this with eating something that your stomach 'can handle', and you'll see that you really need to put some thought into your food shopping.

If you are still unsure then have your partner or friend that's already had a baby, check it for you. They can make sure that you have the right foods on your list. In case you have put 'extra' items on your list, they will make sure they are off the list.

More Top Shopping Tips for Pregnancy

- Don't shop when you're hungry! You may end up with a multi-pack of crisps and fifteen beef burgers in your trolley.
- Why not try shopping online? Lots of the major supermarkets now offer this service. You can take as much time to plan your shopping as you like, you can double check the list and even see how much it's all coming too so that you don't over-spend. Even better, it all gets delivered to your home so there's no carrying bags and boxes and you won't be tempted to chuck that ice-cream in the basket as you go past a display.

Yoga and Exercise in Pregnancy

Yoga and Exercise in Pregnancy

Regular physical movement is just as important as a healthy diet during pregnancy. Contrary to popular belief, exercising during pregnancy is really good for you and baby and can also help you cope better with the physical and mental changes.

During pregnancy, most women suffer from symptoms such as extreme tiredness, backache (among other aches and pains,) and constipation. A simple yoga practice can help you keep all of these niggles at bay.

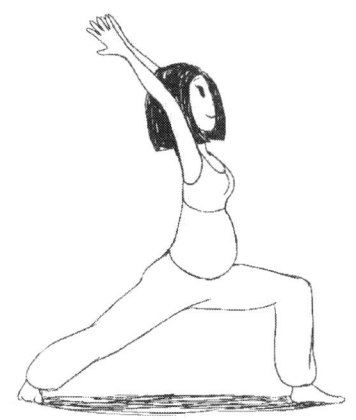

10 Reasons Why You Need to Exercise During Pregnancy

1. Physical exercise releases endorphins that help to lift your mood. If you work out, you will be less prone to pregnancy mood swings. Not to mention the fact that working out helps the body to release of the love drug, my favourite hormone, Oxytocin (read more about this later.)

2. One obvious benefit of exercise during pregnancy, is that it will help you keep a reign on any excessive weight gain.

3. Exercise can also help you avoid developing problems like gestational diabetes or pre-eclampsia during pregnancy.

4. Many women find it hard to get comfortable and to sleep at all at night, during pregnancy, which makes you even more tired the next day. Exercise ensures that you are suitably tired at night and will easily fall asleep (if not

during class!) Yoga makes your body stronger. Strengthening and tonight the body will also help you to prepare for birthing, physically and mentally.

5. Exercise will help increase your stamina, which you will need for birthing and improve your physical well-being before and after baby arrives.

6. Keep fit during pregnancy, through yoga or other low impact exercise, can help prevent or avoid problems such as gestational diabetes, a form of diabetes that sometimes develops during pregnancy.

7. Exercise can also help to prevent the "baby blues" that many new mums experience after the birth of their child.

8. Staying in shape will assist your recovery after the birth of your baby. Always be sure to consult with your midwife or GP before beginning any type of fitness program while you are pregnant.

9. If you work out on a regular basis, you will improve the condition of your joints and muscles. This will make birthing easier, more comfortable and more effective.

10. The long-term effects will also continue after giving birth and will also help you lower your risk of heart disease and many other serious illnesses.

Should Everyone Exercise During Pregnancy?

All pregnant women can and should exercise in moderation, unless there are special circumstances or risks that prevent them from doing so. This should consist of thirty minute sessions, several days a week, if not every day of the week. Yoga philosophy states that six days of practice is more than enough and the seventh day should be a day of rest.

A Pregnancy yoga session with 30 minutes of Asana (yoga postures,) 15 minutes of Pranayama (yogic breathing) and 15 minutes of Savasana (deep relaxation) is just perfect.

Choosing an Exercise Programme for Pregnancy

There are so many fitness programs that are available for pregnant women today, it really depends on what you enjoy, your level of current fitness and what you want to get from your time. Other exercise you can try in addition to your yoga practice, could include walking, swimming, low or no-impact aerobics (done at a mild pace), and Pilates. You should always avoid activities that can put you at a high risk for injury such as horse rising or mountaineering (eek!)

Any sport or exercise that could cause you to be hit in the stomach or where you have to lie on your back for prolonged periods of time, are considered high risk (more about this later.) This is extremely important after the third month, but also in the first trimester, when baby is most vulnerable and the majority of miscarriages happen.

Once your doctor or midwife gives you the go ahead to begin a fitness program, decide on a program that fits both your needs and your schedule. Keep in mind that a 30-minute session is more than enough during pregnancy. 'Little and often' is your pregnancy mantra.

If you have never exercised before, or are finding it difficult to choose an exercise routine that appeals, try a few different types of exercise that are safe for pregnancy, and then decide which you enjoy the most. You may want to incorporate a variety of exercise sessions into your routine, to prevent you from becoming bored or discouraged. If you are taking part in group pregnancy classes, then you will get to meet even more potential mummy friends if you attend a range of classes.

Many of my own clients enjoy coming along to YogaBellies for Pregnancy and AquaBellies (aquanatal yoga) classes. Finding complimentary classes with the same teacher or with a similar ethos, helps prepare you mentally for birthing. With everyone on the same page, you know that you and your baby are safe and secure. Remember also that exercising while you are pregnant, is one of the best things you can do for yourself and your unborn child and that every moment that you spend looking after yourself, is time spent well for baby.

Types of Exercise That Are Perfect During Pregnancy

The best kind of exercise during pregnancy is one that does all of these:
- Keeps you flexible and fit
- Helps you manage weight in a positive and healthy way
- Strengthens your body's muscles for birthing
- Does not cause any sort of stress to you or your baby
- Allows for some 'me time' or relaxation

Clearly=Yoga! ☺ We're biased, I know! Avoid any exercise where you may be at the risk of falling down hard or losing your balance. Examples of these types of exercises are skiing, football, tennis, gymnastics and horse-riding or any HITT. Hold onto the wall if attempting simple standing balances during yoga class.

All yoga and exercise routines will need to be altered as your pregnancy progresses. Stressful exercise is not recommended at all during pregnancy because your body is still adapting to change and you will need more rest. Now is not the time to begin Ashtanga or Bikram yoga, please go along to a class with a qualified pregnancy yoga teacher, to ensure that you are safe and not over-doing it.

I've listed a few different kinds of exercise that you can incorporate into your pregnancy wellness routine, saving (yoga) the best for last! Here are some of the safest forms of exercise for pregnant women.

Pilates

Pilates helps you strengthen your pelvic floor muscles and tummy, but tends not to include a spiritual or relaxing aspect. Your instructor will guide you through a series of physical and breath exercises safe for pregnancy. They may also include breathing practice for child birth but Pilates is very much a 'physical' exercise, without a spiritual or emotional focus.

Walking, Jogging or Running

Walking provides you an excellent cardio workout, without putting you at any kind of risk. You can incorporate walking into your daily routine and it is also completely safe throughout your entire pregnancy. Even if you are unable to get any other form of exercise, you can always go for a walk. Walking can also help you clear your mind and refocus.

Jogging and running are great for getting a good workout and to get your heart pumping but if you weren't a big cardio person before you got pregnant, now is not the time to start. Go for a walk instead and enjoy the view. Listen to a walking meditation recording on your iPhone as you stroll.

Swimming

Swimming is one of the safest forms of exercise during pregnancy. Swimming lets you exercise every muscle groups and safely increases your heart rate. It is safe to swim throughout your pregnancy. Try out our AquaBellies aquanatal and water based yoga classes, if you feel that you are a water baby at heart. More on the brilliant benefits of aqua yoga in pregnancy later.

Aquanatal classes have become very popular lately, and you may find you struggle to get booked into a class. You may want to consider joining one of those if you don't like to swim alone or would like to try prenatal yoga in the water. The routines in AquaBellies classes are good for the joints and can also help ease the swelling from your feet and legs. Who doesn't like to feel weightless when their pregnant? ☺

Weight Training

Lifting free weights can help improve your muscle tone and blood circulation. Unfortunately, as a pregnant woman, there will be a few restrictions placed on your weight-training exercises.

For most of your pregnancy, you shouldn't lift the same weights as you are used to. For one, you should not lift heavy weights, as this could cause harm to your baby. Instead, try using half the weights you used to lift, and increase the repetitions. Small handheld weights are fine, if you are accustomed to weight training and/or are being supervised by a professional.

Before performing any weight training exercises, make sure you consult with your doctor or midwife first. They will be able to tell you what is right for you and what is not acceptable.

Cycling

You may be thinking that cycling is the last thing you would want to do when you are pregnant. The seat will feel uncomfortable, the bumps in the road can hurt and there is the danger of falling. Most of these dangers exist when you are driving a car as well.

If you are a frequent bike rider, there is absolutely no reason for you not to ride your bike from time to time. Just make sure that your seat is well padded, at the correct height and properly angled to accommodate your growing belly. Try to avoid riding uphill, in groups or on the main road, as this can increase the chances of you falling off your bike.

When pregnant, taking your bike for a ride can be very relaxing. It helps strengthen your muscles, improves your breathing and helps calm your body and mind. You also get a chance to enjoy the outdoors. The combined effects help to alleviate emotional stress.

Why YogaBellies Is So Much More Than Exercise for Pregnancy

What is Yoga?

What most people knew to yoga don't know, is that you don't have to get on your yoga mat to do yoga. The way that you live your life is yoga.
Did you know that what you do on the mat (asana) is only one of eight 'limbs' of yoga? But because it's the part you can see, everyone thinks that's all there is to yoga.

Yoga literally means 'Union' and refers to the union of body and mind. So when we practice physical yoga postures, what are actually doing, is a moving meditation.

A Simple Guide to The Eight Limbs of Yoga

The eight limbs of yoga are the basis of all 'Hatha Raja' yoga. Hatha refers to all physical yoga that you practice on your mat, and there is a tendency to call all 'general' yoga classes, hatha yoga.

Raja yoga, is the yoga of the mind, and without this, yoga postures are just another exercise routine. So when we practice yoga, we should always aim to connect, or find union within, our body with our mind. We should try to become fully aware of our physical movements and sensations in the body (especially in pregnancy,) and also of the fluctuations of the mind. By bringing our attention to the breath (Pranayama,) we can calm and soothe the mind, and we will ultimately see benefits to the physical body also.

So What are 'The Eight Limbs?'

Yamas: The Don'ts
These are the things we shouldn't do, such as don't steal or lie or harm things. The aim of the Yamas is to reduce suffering. This could be avoiding those fatty foods in pregnancy or snapping at people because we are tired.

Niyamas: The Do's
These are things personal to you, like contentment and looking within for answers. These are actions and attitudes we should adopt to reduce suffering for us and those around us. In pregnancy, this could refer to the good things that we can do for our body and our baby, such as practicing yoga.

Asanas: Body postures (the yoga that everyone sees!) This limb refers to the act of actually getting on the mat. This is only one of eight limbs, a tiny part of your entire yoga practice! A very important part though and you should aim to practice pregnancy yoga at least three times a week if you can.

Pranayama: Yogic breathing exercises, and the control of Prana (energy.) Pranayama can help cool you, calm you down and help you sleep during pregnancy.

Pratyahara: Control of the senses or withdrawing from the things around (our senses) us, so that we can look inside ourselves for answers and get to know our true selves. It means not always having to react to the crazy world around us. For example, if someone is being bitchy, it could mean being aware of what they are doing but not allowing it to upset you and understanding that they have their own reasons for being a bitch, which are probably unrelated to you. Don't allow it to impact of affect your life.

Dharana: Concentration. This is when we become able to clear the mind to focus on one thing at a time. Try focusing completely on washing the dishes (yes seriously!) It's very, very calming and can help you relax. Now that you are no longer affected by outside influences, you are able to bring your attention to focusing on just one thing at a time.

Dhyana: This is meditation or complete absorption on the object being focused on, or moving beyond the mind. This is perfect contemplation. This is where we can recognize the 'monkey mind' or chatter in our heads, acknowledge it and move past it. We don't need to listen to every little voice that goes running through our head, we are not our thoughts. Dhyana allows us to see things clearly and perceive reality beyond the everyday nonsense that distracts us.

Samadhi: This is what every yogi aspires towards and few reach. It is important to remember that yoga is not goal orientated and it's very much about 'enjoying the journey.' Samadhi, is complete bliss where the mind reaches a state of supreme consciousness. Sometimes we touch upon Samadhi while going about our business...and then we lose it - but just touching it feels lovely :) Samadhi is true yoga or 'union.'

Yoga in Pregnancy

Women endure a lot of physical and emotional stress during pregnancy. Without allowing yourself or learning how to relax fully, you may find pregnancy hard to handle, physically and especially emotionally.

Yoga is incredibly beneficial for pregnant women. As you know, you need to relax your body, calm your mind and breathe deeply during yoga poses. This can help reduce the physical strain on the body and can help significantly during birthing.

If you take yoga classes on a regular basis, just remember to let your instructor know that you are pregnant. It's better to move to a prenatal class as soon as possible. Many yoga teachers who don't have specialist pregnancy training feel very nervous teaching pregnant women and this is not to be advised. Seek out a qualified pregnancy yoga teacher from a reputable school.

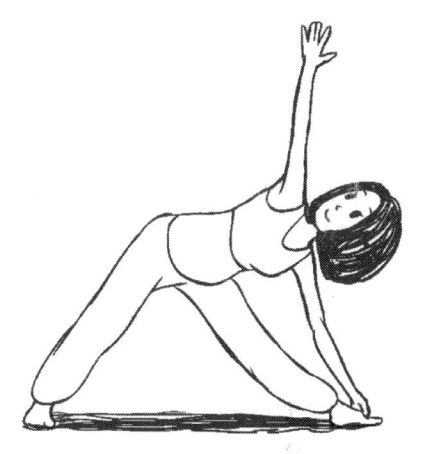

If you are doing yoga for the first time, it is a good idea to join a YogaBellies for Pregnancy class, where 86% of our students have never practiced yoga before. Additionally, contact your midwife/doctor and make sure yoga is safe for you.

Yoga Makes You Happy

The fact is that yoga actually makes you happier. The 'love hormone' Oxytocin helps you to relax and reduces blood pressure and cortisol levels. Yoga is now well recognised as one of the ways to encourage the body to release this amazing hormone and built in anti-stress mechanism.

When the various limbs of yoga are practised, Oxytocin is released. Deep breathing warms the body, and warmth is one of the key elements that allow us to release Oxytocin. By taking the body through the practice of yoga asana (postures) we warm the muscles and joints, make the physical body more comfortable and relaxed. By then continuing the practice with Savasana (deep relaxation) and meditation, we encourage the production of oxytocin even further.

Yoga Helps You Prepare for Birth

Oxytocin is that magical hormone that rushes through the body when we first fall in love. Oxytocin can take us to the dizzy heights of a love sickness that makes food and sleep seem so much less important than looking into the eyes of our new found love.

Some of oxytocin's main functions are preparing the female body for childbirth, stimulating milk production and 'let down' so that baby can nurse, and encouraging the bond between mum and her new-born baby.

The hormone is also plays an important part in sexual arousal and is released when you have an orgasm. It's important in nonsexual relationships too and presence of the hormone has shown to increase trust, generosity, and cooperation. It can also create a nurturing aspect within males and females who are not parents.

Oxytocin helps birthing women through birthing encouraging surges or contractions as well as providing pain relieving endorphins and an altered state of consciousness or bliss (known as birthing land) that makes most of childbirth seems 'dream like' or surreal. As soon as baby is born, it makes mum fall in love in the greatest way possible, with their new-born baby.
In the first few moments after giving birth, a mum receives the largest rush of oxytocin that she will ever experience in her lifetime.
Oxytocin flows between mum and child every time baby is breastfed which encourages bonding and attachment.
During birth we can encourage the release of oxytocin by making sure that mum has privacy, feels safe and comfortable, has a dimmed room and is left in peace. Yogic breathing and practice of adapted Savasana during childbirth can aid the release of this special hormone.

Pranayama Brings You Peace

Yogic breathing (of course!) When the Vagus nerve is inflamed your breathing becomes shallower. Your body has gone into fight or flight mode and you have started to panic. Stop right here and allow yourself to breathe deeply. Pranayama (or yogic breathing) encourages to take time to just stop, and focus on the breath.

Pregnancy and mumhood can bring a lot of huge physical, emotional and environmental changes that can be difficult to adapt to. Taking some time each week to just BREATHE during yoga class, bringing your attention to the breath, focusing on the breath alone, not worrying about anything else, can allow oxytocin to be released and deepen that relaxation. Slow steady breathing is all that you need. Sometimes we get so caught up in 'getting the posture' that we forget to breathe. Check yourself and make sure you ARE actually breathing (you'd be surprised.)

Yoga Warms the Joints and Prevents Injury

It is important to warm the body before undertaking the physical practice of yoga (asana) so as not to damage any joints and to ease the body gently into the postures. This is especially important for pregnant and post-natal women, whose bodies are and have undergone physical stress and growth over a period of time. During the practice of asana and pranayama, the body generates heat and warms the body inside and out. Extra bonus? When we are warm and relaxed, the body releases more oxytocin…

Yoga Soothes and Relaxes

At the end of class, don't just jump up and run out of class. Savasana, deep relaxation at the end of class is your reward for all of your hard effort earlier on. Learn to enjoy the relaxation, be aware of any random thoughts that go through your mind – and just let them go. This is known as 'monkey mind' (What will I have for dinner? What did she mean by that?) – Acknowledge these meaningless thoughts and really take time for yourself – just focus on the life force – the breath. That's all you need to do. And enjoy the scrummy feeling of the copious oxytocin rushing through your body. Sigh.

Yoga Eases Antenatal and Postnatal Depression

In a study of 65 women with depression and anxiety, the 34 women who took a yoga class twice a week for two months showed a significant decrease in depression and anxiety symptoms, compared to the 31 women who were not in the class.

Yoga helps to balance hormones and stabilizes the endocrine system. By practising yogic relaxation techniques, we can balance cortical activities and the nervous and endocrine systems, reducing the body`s reaction to stress. As a result, the body produces less adrenaline, noradrenaline and cortisol, (all stress hormones) and mum feels much more balanced and stress free.

Also, prenatal depression studies indicate clinical depression alleviates by half if only we can talk to a friend who listens to us and oxytocin is shown to increase when we receive empathy. The social aspects of getting out to perinatal yoga classes either before or with baby help mum and baby socialize with other mums around them.

Yoga Helps You Bond with Your Baby

Remember oxytocin is about being personal in ways that give our time together significance and shape moments of laughter and pleasure. Follow the instinct to reach out and strengthen ties with invitations to share together and enjoy your pregnancy and life.

There is ample evidence, that Oxytocin and another hormone known as Vasopressin are critical for the bonding process, especially as it relates to social and reproductive behaviour. Both chemicals help encourage bonding and maternal behaviour.

Six Reasons Why Pregnancy Yoga is Even Better in the Water

There are clearly many physical and psychological benefits that yoga can bring...but most people don't know that there are even more, additional benefits when you take your practice to the pool. Here are a few little known reasons to consider water based movement in pregnancy:

1. Exercising in the water is known for its therapeutic and rehabilitation uses, well designed classes and a motivating instructor will give you a thorough a practice that is just as effective, and possibly even more comfortable, than a land based yoga class.

2. So why is yoga in the water so different to land based practice? Well there are a few reasons for this; hydrostatic pressure; buoyancy and resistance.
   To start with let's look at hydrostatic pressure, a property you cannot benefit from when doing land base yoga. This is the gentle pressure on the body caused by the water when you are in the pool. This increases the deeper into the pool you go, think of your body being gently squeezed by the water. This pressure, along with the movement of the water provides a gentle massaging effect around the body helping with a variety of ailments. As this massaging effect is equal around the body, it assists with circulation and blood pressure by helping the venous return.

3. If you suffer with high blood pressure and the doctor has advised you are safe to take part in yoga, a gentle water based yoga class would be a good way to take part and may help to lower your blood pressure.
   As your circulation is being controlled by the water- there is no added stress on the organs- meaning that your metabolism is still working while you are exercising- this is often why you can feel really hungry after you have been to the pool!

   The gentle pressure temporarily relieves oedema and fluid retention by encouraging the fluid back into the circulatory system (you may need to use the toilet more after your class!). If you are an asthma sufferer (providing chlorine does not have an adverse effect on your asthma), the hydrostatic pressure around your chest while exercising will help to strengthen your respiratory muscles, along with a warm and humid environment should make exercising in the water comfortable.

4. Buoyancy is the "floaty" feeling you get when you enter the water, a feeling of weightlessness that can be well received especially when you are in the later stages of pregnancy. This is also of benefit to those who are overweight or have a problem with their joints.

    This is one of the reasons why water yoga is used in injury rehabilitation, as it reduces the weight being loaded onto the joints, which may be overload for land based yoga and provides temporary relief from aches and pains. Standing chest depth in water can reduce impact on the body by as much as 90%. The buoyancy will change your centre of gravity and therefore your body will be using core muscles to keep you upright, so you will be strengthening important muscles before you even start your yoga! This "floaty feeling" will promote a sense of wellbeing during the relaxation phase of your class and will also help to slow down the pace at which you work at in the water, but don't worry- the resistance will make sure you work just as hard as if you were on land!

5. Resistance- the reason why walking in water seems pretty hard... in fact it is 12 times harder than if you were to walk on land, and the deeper into the pool you are, the stronger the resistance. This water property is what instructors use to create a great workout.

    When not using any water weights you have resistance from every angle, meaning that you are gently toning all areas of your body as you yoga, thus creating a balanced way to improve your fitness. Resistance will also help to slow down your pace, reducing the risk of injury or falls (you can't fall over in the water!). Adding resistance through water depth, water weights or changing your body position will help to provide more of a challenge- therefore the class can be easily adapted for everyone no matter what stage of fitness you are at!

6. The water temperature will keep you feeling comfortable throughout your class, meaning you can work harder during each asana (yogic posture), without necessarily feeling it. The calming effects of the water, combined with your yogic relaxation and breathing techniques will ensure that you

do not leave your class feeling flushed, hot and sweaty but peaceful, invigorated and empowered (albeit slightly hungry!)

Preparing to Practice Yoga During Pregnancy

Pregnancy is not an illness, but that doesn't mean that you won't feel ill or be sick. Many people (myself included,) suffer from extreme sickness, aches and pains and ailments during pregnancy. Your body is undergoing a lot of changes, and you are carrying another life within you – so you can't exactly be reckless about what you do. Even when you are sleeping or sitting still, you are still growing another person, which takes up a whole lot of energy.

During pregnancy, the most important thing you can do is to listen to your body. Don't force yourself beyond your limits or embark on crazy fad diets: this is not the time. That's the key to successful prenatal exercise preparation really: Knowing what you can and can't do.

In this section, we're going to look at how we can best prepare to begin your yoga practice and what safety measures you should be undertaking. This way, your exercise doesn't end up being more of a bane than a benefit.

10 Important Things You Need to Know About Going to A Pregnancy Yoga Class

You will have realized by now that by practicing yoga during pregnancy, can help you work through fluctuating emotions, stay flexible and healthy and become positive about birth and parenting. Here are some things you probably didn't know about yoga for pregnancy and birth...

1. Yoga is not a Cult! People have lots of preconceived ideas about what yoga is and who 'should' practice it. Anyone can do yoga, it helps you become flexible and calm so don't be put off by serene looking photos of people with their legs around their neck

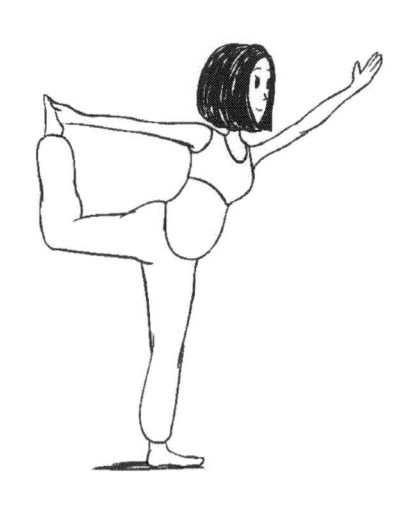

2. it's important to find a yoga teacher that's right for you. If you're new to yoga, YogaBellies classes cater for all levels and make you feel comfortable wherever you are in your pregnancy or your yoga journey. Our teachers are fully qualified in teaching yoga for pregnant women accredited by the IYN, YA and IPTI. If your prospective teacher does not hold a reputable Yoga Teacher Training qualification and specialist training in pregnancy yoga, look elsewhere!

3. Don't worry if you've never tried yoga before. 86% of the mummies who come to YogaBellies pregnancy yoga classes have done very little or no yoga at all before attending. The classes have a nice steady pace and the focus is on practicing at the level you feel comfortable at – everyone will be at a different stage of pregnancy and feel differently so it's important to focus on what feels best for you (and baby.)

4. The most important thing is not to force yourself (or baby,) to do anything you don't feel comfortable with. It's important to listen to your body's signals.

5. If you have practiced yoga before or perhaps have been a dedicated runner or gymnast, prenatal yoga can help you come to terms with the fact that it's no longer just about you. Super fit mums can often find it hard to slow down during pregnancy, but this is just as important as keeping fit. Realizing that you can't do everything the way you used to before you were pregnant is the first lesson in being a parent.

6. A pregnancy yoga class isn't just about keeping fit. Yes, we use especially adapted yoga postures which are safe and beneficial during pregnancy, but at YogaBellies classes you will also learn breathing techniques to use to calm and soothe the mind. These can be used during pregnancy, birth and beyond.

7. We also discuss useful postures to help get baby into the correct position for birth and to help turn a breech baby.

8. We look at postures and positions you can assume during birthing and birth to assist baby's easy entry into the world.

9. At the end of class, we have a lovely deep relaxation and self-hypnosis session, which practiced regularly helps mum remain calm and positive about pregnancy and birth. And yes, we do have lots of sleeping mummies during this part.

10. Pregnancy yoga classes are the perfect place to meet other likeminded mummies. It's so important to meet other mums locally who are at the same stage in life as you and going through the same thing. Peer support will help you through the ups and downs of pregnancy and parenthood

and reassure you that you and your baby are 'normal' and that someone else has probably had the same issue.

Your Pregnancy Yoga Health Checklist

The great thing about yoga, especially pregnancy yoga, is that anyone can do it! A reputable, qualified pregnancy yoga teacher will ALWAYS ask you to complete a health questionnaire before attending class. They will want to make sure that they have all of your vital information, so that they can modify the practice to your needs and safety. If they're not asking these questions, then they don't know or they don't care. Either way, I'd choose another teacher. We're going to cover some of the safety precautions that you should take to minimize your risk of anything untoward happening, the first thing that you should do is ensure that you're not in the way of the more 'general' risks, by checking with your GP or Midwife.

Before you begin a yoga practice, you need to be aware if you fit into any of these categories:
- Have you ever had any pre-existing heart conditions?
- Are you at risk of respiratory conditions or lung disease?
- Do you have diabetes of any kind?
- Do you suffer from high blood pressure or pre-eclampsia?
- Have you previously had a premature birth?
- Have you experienced any physical condition that has prevented you from exercising in the past?
- Have you experienced persistent 2nd or 3rd trimester bleeding?
- Has your water broken (ruptured membranes?)

You probably already know the answers to these questions, but if you are unsure, it's best to check with your midwife. If your answer to all of these questions was a firm 'no', then congratulations, you have little or nothing to worry about, and you should be able to begin your yoga practice with no issues whatsoever.

However, if your answer to any of the questions in the checklist was 'yes', or if you were unsure of the answer, then it is strongly advised that you consult your GP or midwife before you begin your pregnancy yoga practice.

Other relative contraindications/conditions which may need the 'okay' by your GP include:
- Poorly controlled type 1 Diabetes
- Intrauterine growth restriction
- Severe anaemia
- If you are very under or overweight
- If you suffer from chronic bronchitis or are a heavy smoking
- If you have a history of extremely sedentary lifestyle
- If you suffer from poorly controlled hypertension or thyroid disease
- If you are suffering from any kind of acute illness or infection.

This doesn't mean to say that you should stop reading now though.

Over the course of this guide, you'll find that you're able to perform most of the postures and sequences, unless you have a specific condition that prevents you from doing so. Still, it wouldn't hurt to get a professional medical opinion. Better safe than sorry, right? And end of the day, you want to make sure that you're not exposing yourself to any unnecessary risk! Thankfully, yoga is one of the lowest risk forms of exercise for pregnancy and this is why it is so highly recommended. With this initial health checklist out of way, let's move on to some of the basic safety precautions that you should be taking during your pregnancy practice.

Top Tips for Respecting Your Pregnant Body While Practising Yoga

Remember that our golden rule in YogaBellies for Pregnancy is: Listen to your body! Be aware of and respect your limitations. This is your key to a safe and beneficial yoga practice during a pregnancy. A lot of the safety precautions revolve around knowing your limits and not going too far and accepting where you 'are at' are right now. If you've been very active in the past, this can be very difficult to come to terms with, especially at the start of pregnancy, when we don't have a bump. This is when baby is at its most vulnerable.

As you would expect, limits can vary drastically from person to person, depending on how fit they were previously, and how much exercise they're used to.

Don't worry about what size the person on the mat next to you is or what they can or can't do. You and you're your baby are the only people who matter in your practice. Stay focused on your baby and your mat.

1. Listen to your body

Pregnancy is the worst time to overwork or strain your body. There are so many changes going on, that your body will constantly need extra energy reserves. First and foremost, pay attention to your breathing. If you start to feel short of breath, it means that you're pushing your body too far. Your pregnancy yoga teacher will be able to take you through some pregnancy breathing techniques and I've added some later in the book to try at home.

There are a lot of different signs that you're overworking your body, including dizziness, nausea, fatigue, light-headedness, or sudden chills. If you experience any of these things, stop exercising immediately, and take a break. Come into Child's Pose (Balasana) on the ground with your knees wide to accommodate your bump and your forehead on the mat or on a block for support. Should you continue to experience these symptoms, you should seek medical advice.

2. Avoid High Intensity Yoga

Any sort of yoga that involves vigorous jumping or bouncing, is definitely off the table during pregnancy. Remember that when you're bouncing, your baby is going to be bouncing too, and that movement is something that you don't want to put them through! Do NOT force your legs around your head or dive into headstands. Listen to your body – always – and only do what feels right for you.

3. Don't squish your bump!

While some gentle abdominal strengthening exercises are fine, anything that has the potential to cause trauma to your stomach area or womb, is definitely not. Steer clear of things that could potentially injure or harm this delicate area of your body.

In yoga this means no deep twists or postures that restrict the abdomen or squash your bump. If you are asked to do anything like this in a pregnancy yoga class, it's time to find a new class.

4. Stand up straight
Posture is something that is extremely important during a prenatal yoga practice. You should always ensure that your pelvis is gently tilted and your back, straight. Don't lock out or over extend the joints, keep a gentle bend in the knees and elbows at all times.

You should also avoid postures that arch your back, because along with the additional weight of baby, this could end up causing injuries and is not recommended. Bye-Bye Upward Facing Dog!

5. Build it up gently
No matter what level of exercise or yoga practice you may be used to, your pregnancy is making huge changes to your body. You need to accept your new physical limitations and gradually figure out your new level of yoga practice. Remember that this will also change as your pregnancy progresses, your energy levels fluctuate and your bump begins to grow.

6. Stay Cool and Refreshed
One thing that is very important during pregnancy, is making sure that you don't overheat or become dehydrated. Water, water, water. I cannot emphasize enough the importance of water throughout pregnancy. Drink as much as you can because you and baby need it all! Around 8-10 glasses per day is perfect and more if you live in a warm climate.

Avoid exercising outdoors in hot or humid weather, and be sure to drink lots of water at all times. Take water into yoga class and sip at regular intervals. Also, wear light and breathable clothing (yoga pants are perfect) that doesn't cling to your body and cause you to build up more heat than you should.

TOP SAFETY TIP:
Just say NO to Hot Yoga during pregnancy! Hot yoga classes are heated to 40 degrees and a woman's optimal body temperature during pregnancy is 36 degrees. Don't do this to yourself or your baby! Exposing your unborn child to these temperatures can cause birth defects and problems with growth. Even if

you practiced hot yoga before, please avoid for the duration of your pregnancy.

7. Keep off your back and your belly
You should avoid any postures on your tummy or that involve spending a long time on your back after the first trimester. If you'd rather avoid them throughout pregnancy altogether, that's fine too.

If you do exercise on your back, you're opening yourself up to the risk of compressing the Vena cava which carries blood and oxygen to baby, due to the additional pressure. This is why it's recommended that we don't sleep on our backs during pregnancy too. This and the fact that it's very uncomfortable having your organs squished by a big bump of baby.

Basically, if you think about how each posture impacts on baby or your comfort level, you should be able to now determine whether or not it is okay for you to carry it out. If in doubt, you could always consult your own medical expert.

Anyway, we're off to a pretty good start now – and it's time that we delve a little deeper and look at actually getting started on your YogaBellies for Pregnancy practice. Yay!

Getting Started with YogaBellies for Pregnancy

The great news is that starting a YogaBellies for Pregnancy practice, is accessible to everyone. If you've already been practicing regularly, you may that you already know a lot of what I'm about to tell you, but it's always worth going through it again, just in case there's something you missed. Because of your pregnancy, it is all the more important that you have your practice foundations right.

We've covered the things to look out for and what to avoid, and so that should give you a fairly good place to start from. I've also popped together some basic ground rules for beginning a pregnancy yoga practice; the kit and clothes you may need to practice and also why warming up is so important.

The Importance of Warming Up During Pregnancy

Warming up is so important in any form of exercise as it limbers up your body, gets your blood flowing, and ensures that your body is well prepared for whatever exercise you're planning to undertake. Jumping straight into a yoga practice, without making sure that your body is ready, is a recipe for disaster.

If your muscles are tight and tense, you could end up injuring yourself. During pregnancy, our body releases Relaxin which allows the joints to soften, which means we can easily hyper extend. If you find yourself a lot 'bendier' than usual and able to suddenly get your legs around your head, beware! Relaxin allows us to reach yogic heights we could never before, but this can lead to over extension and damage over time. Basically – you don't want any of this to happen.

Warming up properly means that this won't happen. Bearing this in mind, let's walk you through some of the basics of a good yoga warm up so that you can get started at home.

Warming Up the Yogic Way

Warming up is really, part of your practice itself, and it should be carried out right at the start of every yoga practice.

About 5 to 10 minutes of warming up is ideal. During that time, the bulk of it should be spent on stretching your various muscle groups. Naturally, the inclination may be to focus on the big muscle groups, and the ones that your workout is going to use most – but really, you should try to encompass as many muscles as possible.

One way to go about stretching effectively is to start at your head, and work your way down. What this means is that you should start with your neck muscles, then releasing the muscles of the face and the jaw. Allow the tongue to lie limp in the mouth. Let l all go, make sure you release all tension.

You can warm up from standing in Tadasana (mountain pose) or even sitting in Sukkhasana (easy pose or simple cross legs.) Move on to your shoulders, upper arms, chest, lower arms, torso, back, and waist. Neck and shoulder rolls, Garundasana (eagle) arms and Namaskar (reverse prayer) arms are nice places to start. Add in some wrist circles too, just make sure everything is flowing and ready to move. I've written more about these in the pre-written sequences section.

Move further down the body to your hips and pelvis and abdomen, hamstrings, upper legs, and calves and then ankles. Pelvic rolls and tilts, gentle open twists, tiny dancer and ankle rolls are prefect here.

Each of the practices in this book, incorporates a gentle yogic warm up as part of the routine, and this can be seated or standing. A Mama Salutation, my pregnancy adaptation of the Sun Salutation (Surya Namaskara) is a warm up and a full practice in one. It's an easy sequence to remember and learn and I always say to my students that ten rounds per day, will keep you fit as a fiddle, healthy, alert and work every muscle in your body.

No Pain, No Gain = Nonsense

When you are stretching, a common mistake that people make is to stretch until they feel slight pain. Frankly, this 'no pain, no gain' logic is crazy and never applies in a yoga practice – especially during pregnancy. You should never push yourself so far that it actually hurts you.

Instead, gauge your limit, and be sure to stretch – but not overstretch. Overstretching to the point where it is painful, can actually cause muscle tears, which are the last things that you want during pregnancy! Remember all of that Relaxin rushing around your body, making you think that you are the incredible stretchy woman. Also, when you're stretching you should be doing so in slow and measured motions. Don't 'bounce' or 'jerk' your motion.

Some people like to include a quick, slow paced cardiovascular exercise in their warm up stage, just to get the blood flowing. This isn't entirely necessary, but it isn't harmful either, and could help bridge the gap between your warm up stage and your full practice. Again, a Mama Salutation or similar Vinyasa (yoga flow) practice is perfect for this. A few rounds will have you hot, happy and ready to practice.

Creating your Pregnancy Yoga Space

Pregnancy is a time of focus, on yourself and on the little person growing inside of you. Yoga is also a time for reflection and relaxation and your practice should ideally be quiet, with no interruptions. If you have other children or toddlers running around, this is not always possible, so it could be best to set a specific time aside each week and to attend a class with a qualified pregnancy yoga teacher.

Sacred Space

If you're going to practice at home (and you should,) or in addition to a led yoga class, then you should try to set aside a 'sacred' space just for yoga and meditation. This can be your special place, for you and baby to bond, stretch and relax together. If you don't have a spare room to use, even a corner of the living room or bedroom is perfect. Perhaps create a mini altar, with fresh flowers, crystals, candles and incense. Perhaps place your baby's scan photo on the altar as a focus for your practice. This doesn't have to be an actual 'altar' and can be a shelf, table or clear space on the floor. Decorate as you wish, and use this as your Drishti or focus, during your time to practice yoga.

Making a specific time and a special place for your yoga is essential for maintaining a regular practice. Choose a place that is warm and where there is enough room for you to move freely. All you need is a space the size of your yoga mat, as you need never move outside of the mat space during your practice. It's great to set up a routine and to practice at the same time every day, the best times being first thing in the morning or just before bed.

Building a Regular Practice

A regular practice is the best way to experience the many benefits of yoga and it's through your practice, that yoga becomes integral to your life. Allow up to 2 hours after a meal before you begin your practice, if possible. That said, if moving around makes you nauseous, feel free to take biscuits or cheesy Wotsits into class to alleviate the feelings as required.

Think about how much time you have to practice every day (be realistic) and how many times a week. If you can even manage ten minutes every day, this is enough to keep you flexible, well and focused. Begin your session with some pranayama or a short meditation, some mama salutations to warm up, moving onto standing postures, then seated postures, meditation and finishing by relaxing in side-lying corpse pose or Savasana.

Your Pregnancy Yoga Kit

The good news is that you probably have everything you need around the house already. You don't have to break out your credit card, just be comfortable and safe.

Be sure to wear loose fitting and light clothes that don't restrict you or cause your body to overheat. It's not a fashion show so please don't stress. You can buy lovely flowy yoga pants on eBay or from retailers such as Asquith, who over bamboo yoga clothing for pregnancy. You can even buy pregnancy yoga pants and leggings in shops such as New Look, Top Shop and River Island now. Purchase a comfortable and well cushioned yoga mat. When you are pregnant you will need extra support, so make sure that you don't buy one that's too thin. A 6mm thickness is perfect for a pregnancy yoga practice.

You should also have a block and a strap (this can be an old tie and a book if needs be.) Have a couple of cushions for supporting you in reclined postures and also a blanket and socks for Savasana, as you will cool down very quickly at the end of your practice and you don't want to be distracted by the cold.

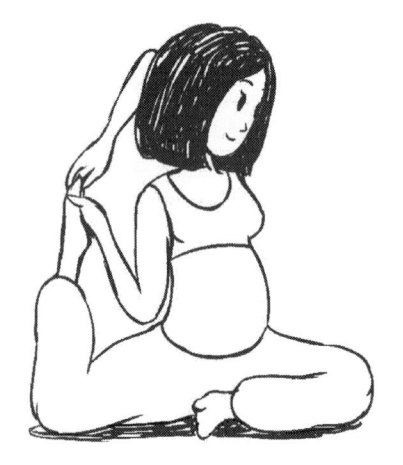

Pranayama (Breathing) for Pregnancy

Yogic breathing (or Pranayama) has huge benefits for everyone, especially during pregnancy and childbirth. Pranayama helps to relax you if you are feeling, tired, anxious or stressed. It can also revitalize you and give you more energy when you feel that you just can't keep going.

Yogic breathing is a great place to start if you've never practiced yoga before. So before you even get in the mat, or if you feel too icky to practice, you can take some time to try out these breathing techniques. Pranayama can help when our thoughts start racing (especially in the middle of the night) and you just can't 'turn off' that monkey mind. So it's great for helping you to sleep too.

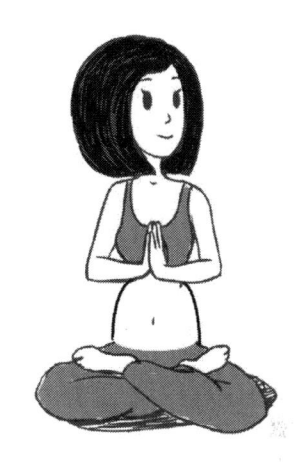

Pranayama also send oxygen and nutrients to the brain cells and releases lots of the yummy Oxytocin that we've been talking about. Deep breathing pumps spinal fluid to the brain; prevents any build-up of toxins in the lungs and stimulates the pituitary gland. Who knew breathing could do so much?

Top Tips for Pregnancy Pranayama

In this guide, we are focusing on your pregnancy and not specifically your actual birth, so let's look at some great YogaBellies for Pregnancy breathing practices you can make use of now.

Before you begin with any pranayama, there are some important things you need to remember, even if you are a seasoned yogini and practice yogic breathing regularly.

- No breath retention (Khumbak) or holding the breath when practicing pranayama pregnant. This can restrict the oxygen supply to your little one and we do NOT want to do that.
- Avoid pumping breaths like Kapalabhati also. If you don't know what this is, don't worry, just follow the Pranayama exercises in this guide or with your YogaBellies for Pregnancy teacher and you will be just fine.
- Whether you are practicing yoga or just going about your everyday activities, try to slow down the breath and make it more even. Deep breathing is fantastic for baby. Keep it natural though, we're not suggesting that you sit in the office like Darth Vader frightening your co-workers. The breath should always be voluntary NOT forced. Take it easy, tune into your body and go with the flow of the breath.

Beautiful Breathing for Pregnancy

I've included three very useful Pranayama practices that are safe and great for pregnancy.

1. Ujjayi breathing: The perfect Darth Vader style breath to use during your pregnancy yoga practice.
2. Nadi Shodana: A cooling breath and great for promoting emotional and mental balance.
3. Brahamarri Humming Bee: Helps keep you alert and upbeat. Baby will love this too and will probably start to kick when you do this.

Ujjayi Breathing (oo-Ji-EE)

Ujjayi breathing, or Darth Vader breath as it's commonly known for its ominous sound, is commonly used in pregnancy yoga classes and during most yoga practice. In a regular (non-pregnancy) yoga class, it is used to soothe the body and mind, create internal heat within the body which allows fluid movement and stretching. Ujjayi breathing also provides a great point of focus during your actual yoga practice, encouraging your asanas (postures) to flow into a moving meditation. Ujjayi breath in a pregnancy yoga practice has all of the same benefits, in addition to providing breath awareness and practice for childbirth.

How to do it:
1. Come into simple cross legged position, with your spine straight and tall.
2. Place your hand in front of your mouth (but not touching it) and take a deep breath in through your nose.
3. On your exhale, open your mouth and expel the air with a "haaaaahhh" sound as though you are fogging a mirror. This sound, created by the slight restriction in the back of your throat is the ocean (or Darth Vader) sound that you will make during ujjayi breath.
4. Allow a smile to gently form on the lips. This helps to open the back of the throat. Do not clench the jaw.
5. Take another inhale through the nose, and on the exhale close your mouth and exhale through your nose. Try to create the same sound in the back of your throat.
6. Now try and create the same sound on your inhalation (this is usually difficult at first and may take practice).
7. Continue to inhale and exhale throughout your yoga practice or as required.

Nadi Shodana (nah-dee shod-an-a) - Alternate Nostril Breathing

The breathing technique helps calm the mind, cool the body and helps you to prepare for meditation. This practice also helps to store and control Prana (vital energy.) Nadi Shodana cool you down on a hot day and also strengthens and cleanses the entire respiratory system.

Because our breathing naturally alternates between the two nostrils, changing roughly every 2 hours, practicing Nadi Shodana helps balance the two elements: The right represents the hot sun and the left is the cool moon.

How to do it:
1. Sit in easy pose or simple cross legs. Make sure your back is straight and your head and spine erect. Position your left hand in chin mudra (index finger

touching middle finger) and your right hand in Vishnu mudra extend. Take 2 or 3 deep breaths here and close your eyes.
2. Inhale deeply through both nostrils and bring the right hand to the nose and cover the right nostril with your right thumb.
3. Exhale slowly through the left nostril slowly for 8 seconds. Less if this is uncomfortable.
4. Now inhale through the left nostril for around 4 seconds. Again, reduce this if you have to.
5. Exhale through the right nostril for 8 seconds.
6. Now inhale through the right nostril for 4 seconds.
8. Continue to repeat the same process for at least three rounds up to 10 rounds a day.
This is a modified version of Nadi Shodana with no breath retention. Remember to never hold the breath while pregnant.

Brahamarri (brahm-ar-ee) - Humming Bee Breath

Brahmarri is the 'humming bee' breath. Brahmarri is thought to be soothing and nourishing for pregnant mothers and babies.

How to do it:

1. Bring yourself into Sukkhasana (easy pose or cross legged) and take a few deep breaths here.
2. Take the hands to the ears, elbows pointing out.
3. Inhale through both nostrils and then exhale making a humming sound like a bee.
4. Allow the length of the breath to extend naturally and without force, humming until the body is empty of breath and then inhaling again
4. Practice for 5 minutes each day.

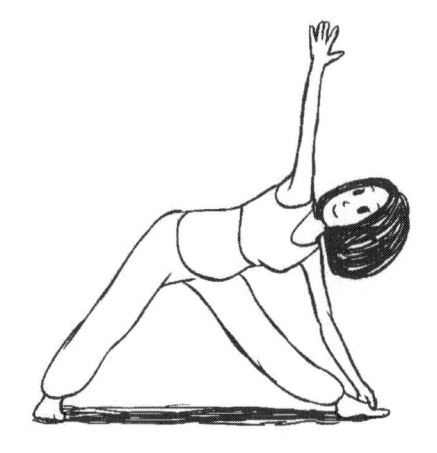

YogaBellies for Pregnancy Meditation... Meet your Baby

Meditation is another aspect of yoga practice which is very important. In fact, the whole purpose of practicing yoga postures, is so that we can sit comfortably in meditation. Only practicing physical yoga without pranayama (yoga breathing) and meditation, in addition to the right livelihood associated with yoga, is really just aerobics.

The dictionary definition of the word Meditation from the Oxford Reference Dictionary 1992:

"To think deeply and quietly; to do this in religious contemplation."

You don't have to be religious or even a yogi to meditate and it is not associated with any religion. There are many forms of meditation and it hold many connotations for yogis and those new to yoga alike. I have included a short baby bonding meditation for you to try, assuming that you are either new to meditation, or at least new to pregnancy.

Why Should I Meditate During Pregnancy?

- Meditation helps to calm the mind, reduce anxiety and anger and helps to eliminate stress. Avoiding these emotions is important for mum and baby's wellbeing during pregnancy and so meditation can be an important tool.
- Meditation affects the body on a deep level and allows us to connect to a healthier state of mind and body.
- It can help us move towards becoming more patient, more aware and more tolerant: all fantastic skills that you're going to need as a new parent!

Here is a gentle introduction to yoga meditation for pregnancy. Just now, you are probably thinking and wondering about your unborn baby all of the time, so it makes sense to focus on your baby while meditating.

During this baby bonding meditation, you will connect with your baby and begin to communicate with them in utero. It will help you to feel completely relaxed and will encourage you to enjoy your pregnancy.

How to Do It

Find a comfortable position, in Hero Pose (Virasana,) Easy Pose (Sukkhasana or simple cross legs) or in Padmasana (Full Lotus.) You can meditate lying down, but when you are pregnant there is a tendency to fall asleep. Use a blanket to cover your knees or around your shoulders to keep you warm and dim the lights if you can. Just as with Pranayama, it's great if you can have a quiet space to practice, but if you don't, just bring your attention to the background noise and then let it go. Keep bringing your attention back to your breath.

1. Inhale deeply and then exhale slowly, a nice long extended exhale. Close your eyes softly and allow yourself to relax completely into your breath and into your body.
2. Take another deep inhale and then exhale slowly to the count of 8.
3. Continue to take a gentle inhale and a long extended exhale. On the in-breath, bring your awareness to your expanding abdomen and as you breathe out, become aware of air leaving your abdomen. As you breathe in, visualize all of your energy as a beautiful pink glow, going down to your belly and to your baby as you inhale. Imagine the pink fuzzy glow warming your body on the in-breath.
4. Now it's time to speak with your baby. Tell them: "I Love you." Take this moment to talk to your baby, introduce yourself to them and tell them what life will be like with their new family. Taker this time to get to know your new baby. Tell them all about their mama and how much fun you are going to have together. Tell baby how excited you are about the pending birth and how you are going to work as a team to make it a calm, peaceful and speedy experience.
5. Continue to breath and as you do, visualize the beautiful pink fuzzy glowing energy surrounding you and your baby now. This energy is protecting you both. Relax into your breathing and allow the flow of pink energy to travel around you and your baby's body.
6. Breathing naturally in rhythm now. Allow yourself to relax and rest. Be at peace with your baby and just become aware of their essence. You and

your baby are safe, happy and loved. You can spend as little or as much time as you like meditating. When you are ready, just open your eyes and gently return to your normal daily activities.

The First Trimester and Getting to Know Your Pregnant Self

The first trimester is very important for you and baby and this is when your pregnancy is at its most vulnerable. Since, not all women follow their menstrual cycle or take note of every time they have intercourse, you may not be sure of your exact date of conception. That is why most women find out that they are pregnant only after the first month of pregnancy.

If you take a note of the dates when you think baby was conceived, this will help your doctor or midwife determine your baby's due date. Remember that a due date is actually a 'due month.' Baby will not expire on the due date that you are giving, this is simply an estimate. Two weeks before and two weeks after this date are perfectly normal times to give birth, so try not to become too fixated on that 'date.' Baby will arrive when they are ready.

As I said before, the first trimester is the most critical and when we are most vulnerable, in every pregnancy. Your baby will be developing all of its vital organs like its lungs, brain and heart, at this time. Lots of women think that self-care and nutrition are not as important at this time, as they are 'only a little bit pregnant,' when nothing could be further from the truth.

This section will take you through basic pregnancy nutrition and recommended foods for the first trimester, and some meal plans for guidance for each month. I've explained what is happening with mum and baby during this trimester and also provide some Ayurvedic top tips. There are some YogaBellies for Pregnancy routines at the end of the section, suitable for all levels of yoga practice, if you are ready to get physical.

What's Happening with Mum and Baby in the First trimester?

Looking after your body and mind in this trimester will impact on your entire pregnancy, and on your baby's vital growth and development, even after birth. I know that until you have a bump, especially if you are lucky enough not to suffer from sickness in early pregnancy, you sometimes you may even forget that you are pregnant. Be aware now, of everything that you eat, say and do for yourself and baby, starting now.

First Month

From the moment of conception until the end of the first trimester, a whole lot is happening for both of you. Baby is still in a jelly-like state until the end of the first few weeks. The zygote begins to divide immediately after conception and travels down the fallopian tube and embeds in the thick, cozy lining of the womb where it links up with your blood vessels. This is where fertilization and implantation occur. Even at this early stage, your baby's brain, heart and spinal cord are beginning to form. Baby is teeny tiny at only 1/25th of an inch long.

Second Month
In the second month, your baby is floating peacefully in a fluid-filled sac and it has a simple brain, spine and central nervous system. Their digestive and respiratory systems are beginning to develop. The baby's heart begins to beat, the neural tube along the baby's back closes and the umbilical cord appears.

In Ayurveda, the heart is considered to be the 'seat of consciousness.' Baby's heart is connected to your heart through arteries and through the placenta. It is through this incredible link, that baby can sense your emotions and feelings at this time. Baby is roughly 2 inches long at this time.

Third Month
In the third month, all of baby's senses, organs and limbs are present. Baby now has completely formed limbs including teeny fingers and toes. Their heart has started beating and is circulating blood. Baby is beginning to move and their sex may even be apparent at this stage. Little fingernails and toenails appear around this time too.

A very important (and lovely) piece for Ayurvedic advice for the third month, is that mum should be looked after and given anything she desires (double whoop!) in order to prevent any mental or physical suffering your unborn child. It is very important to pay close attention to your cravings and desires at this time, and to try to stay positive, happy and focused on your beautiful little person to be.

It is said in Ayurveda, that is mother is overwhelmed with sadness or anxiety during pregnancy, then this will have a negative impact on baby and they will inevitably feel it too. Bonding with baby in utero and your levels of overall happiness and contentment help to ensure proper development of the baby's physical heart and also soul. Baby is around 3 inches long and weighs 4/5 of an ounce.

Recommended Foods for the First Trimester

During the first trimester, people may not know that you are pregnant. You will gain some weight, but you don't really need to be eating a lot of extra calories. You may look as if you have gained a few pounds, but people probably won't realize that you are pregnant yet. You will start to lose the shape of your waist and may just feel like a bit of a blob for a while. Try to increase your daily calorie intake by around 200-300 calories: don't break out the pies and the kit-kats!

In the first trimester, you should be eating foods that are rich in folates. These foods contain folic acid, which assists in the baby's growth and proper development. Aside, from eating folate-rich foods, you should also take a daily supplement of folic acid. Folic acid helps with the baby's physical and neural tube development.

Examples of folate-rich foods you can be eating are oranges, broccoli, eggs, bran flakes, and asparagus. This should ideally start up to six months before conception, or as soon as you can. If you feel too nauseous to take tablet supplements another option is to try a liquid pregnancy multivitamin. These can be hard to find in the pharmacy, but a quick look on line and you will find a lot. Even though the first trimester is crucial for the baby's growth, it's possible that you are feeling too nauseous to eat anything. Snacking was my saviour during this period and I always had a healthy snack to hand (and sometimes cheesy wotsits too.) Vitamin B6 can also help to ease any queasiness or morning sickness. Some food packed with Vitamin B6-rich include wholegrain toast, oily fish such as salmon and bananas.

Pregnancy Smoothie Power!

I will mention smoothies quite a bit in the upcoming pregnancy meal plans, so I thought it would be a good idea, to talk a little about these. All smoothies, especially green smoothies and eating healthy are great things to do while pregnant. Do NOT attempt a full-blown cleanse or detox during pregnancy, this

is not a good idea for you or baby. If your body begins to detox during pregnancy, then toxins will exit your body any way they can–including through the placenta and into your baby.
If you've never attempted a smoothie before, I've included three recipes that are great pregnancy and super easy to make. You can make up your own combinations with your own preferences, just try to stick to our guidelines on safe fruits:

Yoga Baby Power Green Smoothie

1 cup raspberries
1 cup strawberries
1 banana
2 cups almond milk, unsweetened
2 cups Swiss chard, fresh
1-2 tablespoons flaxseed

Yoga Mama Power Smoothie

10 ounces' fresh fruit smoothie
1/2 cup plain Greek yogurt
2 tablespoons chia seeds
1 1/2 cups frozen mango
2 cups fresh spinach

Pink Power Pregnancy Smoothie

1 cup of strawberry chunks
1 kiwi cut into chunks
A splash of lemon juice
1/2 cup ice
1/2 cup milk

Meal Plans for the First Trimester

Making a meal plan from day one, helps you stick to your healthy resolve.

In the first month you should try to always eat wholesome food. You should aim to have at least 2 glasses of milk everyday throughout your pregnancy. In the first month, it should be consumed at room temperature, first thing in the morning. If you still feel nauseous or are vomiting, you can try flavouring milk with cardamom or dry ginger. Your breakfast should consist of mainly sweet, cold and semi-solid foods at this time.

Here are three meal plans, perfect for each month of the first trimester. Be sure to mix them up a little, these are just examples.

First Month

Meals Days	Breakfast	Lunch	Dinner
Monday	1 glass of fresh fruit smoothie or milk. A bowl of Porridge made with 1 tbsp. apple puree and pinch of cinnamon.	1 Banana. Smoked Chicken, Avocado and Asparagus Salad.	Chicken and rice with carrots, tomatoes and green veggies
Tuesday	1 glass fruit smoothie or cold milk. Spinach omelet. Greek yogurt, ginger and chopped fresh fruit.	A bunch of grapes. Baked potato with cheddar cheese.	Chicken cacciatore with brown rice.
Wednesday	1 glass of Fresh fruit smoothie or glass of cold milk. A bowl of bran flakes with milk and a sliced banana.	Roast chicken with potatoes, carrots and broccoli. Fresh fruit salad or fruit smoothie.	Sausage and apple casserole

Thursday	1 cup of green tea and/or glass of cold milk. A bowl of Porridge made with milk, flavored with 1 tbsp. of fresh berries.	A bowl of ripe papaya. Feta salad with couscous.	Pasta with garlic bread.
Friday	A glass of cold milk. A boiled egg with or without whole grain toast.	A slice of melon. Lentil soup.	Lamb chops with potatoes, peas and broccoli.
Saturday	A glass of cold milk. A bowl of Greek yogurt mixed with 1 tbsp. chopped dried fruit and muesli.	1 kiwi. Watercress and Salmon salad.	Creamy fish pie salmon and haddock with Asparagus.
Sunday	A glass of cold milk. Scrambled eggs on toasted bagel.	1 apple. Broccoli and pea soup with a crusty whole-wheat roll.	Tofu and butternut squash flan.

Second Month

In the second month, remember to keep up your water intake, aiming for at least 8 glasses of water every day.

Meals Days	Breakfast	Lunch	Dinner
Monday	A fruit smoothie or milk. 2 boiled eggs.	1 Banana. Smoked Chicken with Avocado Salad.	Grilled pork chop with sweet potato mash, asparagus and green beans.

Tuesday	A yoghurt drink or milk. A bowl of bran flakes with milk and sliced banana.	1 orange. 1 handful of grapes. Broccoli and pea soup.	Baked salmon with potatoes, and broccoli.
Wednesday	A fruit smoothie or milk or milk. 2 slices of wholegrain toast and a boiled egg.	A bunch of grapes. Lentil soup.	Brown rice chicken and mushroom risotto.
Thursday	A cup of green tea or milk. A bowl of Greek yogurt mixed with ginger, chopped mango and 1 tbsp. granola.	1 Apple. Minestrone with a crusty whole grain roll.	Spanish chicken with couscous.
Friday	1 glass of fresh fruit smoothie or milk. A Bowl of muesli with plain yoghurt and chopped apple.	A slice of melon. Baked potato with cherry tomatoes, grated cheddar cheese, chopped cucumber and spring onions	Chicken and Orange casserole
Saturday	1 glass of fresh fruit smoothie or milk. 2 scrambled eggs with Spinach and wholegrain toast.	Chopped mango and pineapple. Carrot, tomato and green veggie salad.	Masma Rasa (meaty soup)
Sunday	1 glass of fresh fruit smoothie or milk. A bowl of porridge with 1 tsp of honey and	Roast beef with roasted parsnips and carrots, with peas Fresh fruit salad or fruit smoothie.	Griddled chicken breast with mango salsa, new potatoes and peas

	fresh fruit chopped.		

Third Month

Try this Ayurvedic tonic in the third month. Take room temperature milk and add honey. Mix the following together in these quantities:

- 2tsps of ghee
- 1tsp of honey
- 1 cup of luke warm milk.

Meals Days	Breakfast	Lunch	Dinner
Monday	A fruit smoothie or milk. A bowl of wholegrain cereal with milk and 1 tbsp. of chopped fresh fruits.	1 Orange. Masma Rasa (meaty soup)	Baked salmon with potatoes and broccoli.
Tuesday	1 glass of fresh fruit smoothie or milk. Toasted whole grain bagel with cheddar cheese and sliced tomato.	1 Apple. Baked potato with spring onions and grated cheddar cheese.	Creamy fish pie of haddock and salmon with peas.
Wednesday	1 glass of Fresh fruit smoothie or milk. Greek yogurt with ginger, with dried	1 Pear. Smoked chicken and avocado salad with rye crackers.	Pork with a baked potato and mushroom, low-fat crème fraiche sauce.

	fruit and nuts and 1 tbsp. of muesli.		
Thursday	A fruit smoothie or milk. 2 slices of wholegrain toast with 1 hardboiled egg	A slice of melon. Pumpkin soup and a crusty roll.	Baked salmon with sweet potato wedges and corn on the cob.
Friday	A yoghurt drink. Bran flakes with milk and sliced banana.	1 kiwi. Egg, watercress and tomato baguette.	Masma Rasa (meaty soup) Stewed apples.
Saturday	Fruit smoothie or milk. Muesli with chopped fruit.	1 banana. Lentil soup.	Turkey breast strips, green beans and peas.
Sunday	1 glass of fresh fruit smoothie or milk. Toasted whole wheat bread with banana.	Roasted pork with green beans. Fresh fruit salad or fruit smoothie.	Tofu and butternut squash flan.

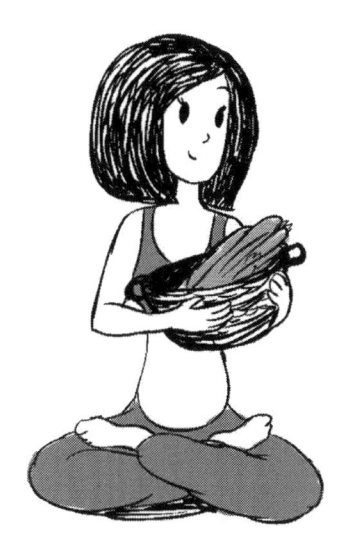

YogaBellies in the First Trimester

If you have an existing yoga practice, it's possible that you didn't know you were pregnant and/or just continued as normal. Although this is okay to do if you have a strong practice, there are still certain postures and types of yoga you should now be avoiding (see the section at the start of your yoga practice.) I have included some simple yoga routines at the end of this section to get you started with a pregnancy yoga practice in trimester one, if you wish to do so. Remember, you may still be feeling nauseous, so don't rush it or force yourself. Listen to your body (I will keep saying it!) and do what feels right. Perhaps start trying out some of the basic postures I have outlined or focusing on meditation and yogic breathing.

Remember that unless you are an experienced yoga practitioner with an existing practice, you should not undertake yoga until 14-16 weeks' gestation. I highly recommend if you are completely new to yoga, then you should join a YogaBellies for Pregnancy class or if you can't commit to a class, try our YogaBellies for Pregnancy DVD or the mini YogaBellies for Pregnancy Practices that I've included at the end of this chapter

Five Basic Pregnancy Yoga Postures to Get You Started

Here are some easy to try yoga postures for you to try at home. Work with these if you are completely new to yoga and when you feel comfortable and confident, move onto the sequences.

Cat Curls (Bidalasana): Bidalasana helps relieve lower back pain and to release the length of the spine, a common problem during pregnancy. Get down on your hands and knees with hands placed directly under shoulders and knees under the hips.
Inhale and lift your heart, stretch back through your tail and concave your spine.
Exhale and roll your spine, lowering the head, pressing through the hands back to straight back. Cat Curls in pregnancy differ from your normal cat curl as we don't curl the abdomen towards the floor, after curling up we simply return to flat back or table top. Repeat following your breath – Inhale as your curl the spine up and exhale back to flat back.

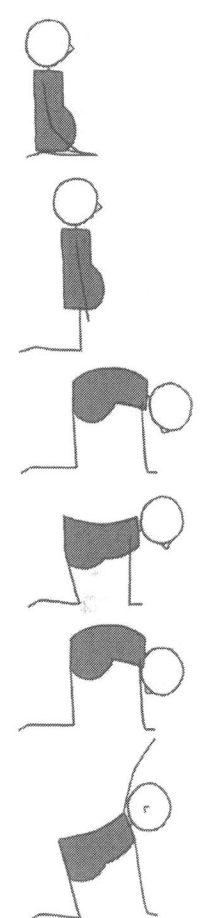

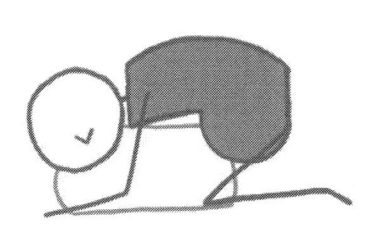

Childs Pose (Balasana): From any kneeling position, sit your tail back toward your heels. Take the knees as far apart as you need to, to make your bump comfortable. Sit back as far as is comfortable and rest your head toward the mat. If you can't reach your head to the mat, rest your chin on your hands. You can stack your fists and rest your forehead there or use a block if you can't quite get down. Otherwise, you can stretch your arms out long in front of you and lower your head all the way to the mat. Avoid Balasana if you are suffering from sciatica.

Bound Angle Pose (Baddha Konasana) - Baddha Konasana is a classic pregnancy yoga posture and is excellent for helping to open up the hips and pelvis in preparation for birth. This is a posture that be practised at night while reading a book or watching TV and is especially important for the later stages of pregnancy in the third trimester.
Sit on your mat with the soles of the feet together.

Bring your heels as close to the groin as possible and pull the shoulder back and down away from the ears to straighten the spine. Hold the feet with the hands and (with a straight spine) begin to gently bend forwards from the hips – only as much as is comfortable – please do not squish your baby! Remember to breathe in and out through the nose.

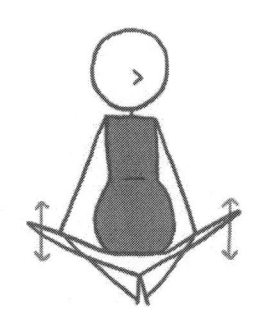

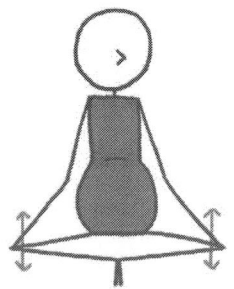

Downward Facing Dog (Adho Mukkha Svanasana): Downward dog can be practised with feet wider apart than normal to accommodate your bump, although ideally no further apart than hip width. Placing the lags and bottom against the wall can help support you also.

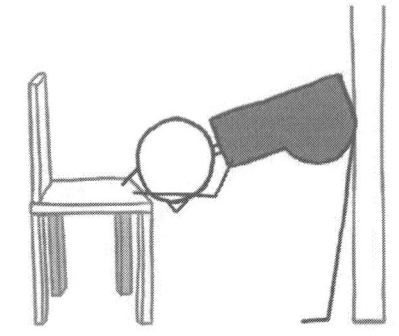

Push into the palms of the hands and pull up on the hip bones. When and if ready, takes the heels to the mat. Its fine to keep the knees bent when pregnant and focus on stretch from hands to hips, lengthening the back.
Only hold any inversion for 5 seconds during pregnancy and if you feel dizzy or nauseous at all, come back down onto the mat and into child pose and relax.

Yoga Squats (Malasana): Squats are great for building strength and stamina during pregnancy and in preparation for birth. Many women like to squat while birthing. As you get bigger in pregnancy, use props such as blocks, bolsters or a Rolled up blanket to rest your bottom on. Focus on relaxing and letting your breath drop deeply into your belly. Stand facing the back of a chair with your feet slightly wider than hip-width apart, toes pointed outward.

Squat towards the floor as though you were going to sit down in a chair. Contract the abdominal muscles, lift your chest, and pull the shoulders back and down. Most of your weight should be toward your heels. This can be done against the wall for support. Remember to avoid wide legged postures if suffering from pelvic girdle pain or PSD.

YogaBellies Mama Salutation

The Mama Salutation, is a pregnancy adapted sun salutation that I put together to accommodate all mamas. It's a great warm up for the rest of your practice or an entire practice in itself.

Standing Tall
Take your feet a little wider apart in Tadasana (Mountain Pose,) than you normally would to accommodate your bump as it grows. Don't take your hand above your head if you are suffering from High Blood Pressure, just rest them in front of your heart in prayer pose.

Forward Bending
Always take a slight bend in the knees as you fold forward and don't stress about touching the ground. Again, watch out for your bump! If bending forward makes you feel dizzy or sick, just bend the knees slightly and bring your elbows to your knees, and hands together in prayer position. You can rest here and then pop onto all fours when it's comfortable to do so.

Downward Facing Dog
You don't have to come into Downward Facing Dog pose (Adho Mukkha Svanasana,) if your bump feels too heavy or you are just uncomfortable. You can continue with your Cat-Cow pose (Bidalasana) or come into Child's Pose.

Stepping Forward
If you have an existing yoga practice, you may be used to jumping forward and back in your sun salutations. Bouncing is not a good idea during pregnancy, so just gently step or nudge your way back to the front of the mat. It may not be graceful and that's cool too.

Legs Up the Wall Pose
Pop a block or cushion under your hips to elevate them slightly in Viparitta Kirana, meaning you are not lying straight down on your back.

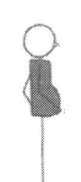

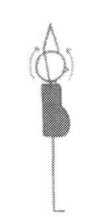

Stand in Mountain pose with feet hip width apart. Keep a gentle bend in the knees. Inhale as you bend elbows and raise arms above head, hands crossing body as you do so.

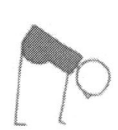

Exhale and bend forward as far as is comfortable. Bend knees if need to and take hands to knees, shins or floor. Use props as desired.

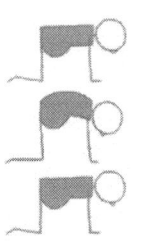

Come onto all fours with flat back. Inhale and curl the back upwards, look towards your bump. Exhale and back to flat back. Repeat x 10.

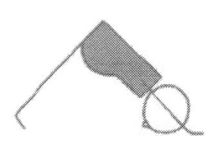

Take feet about 1 meter apart, R foot 90 degrees and back foot at 45. Raise arms in prayer and look towards .

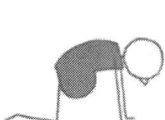

Come back to all fours and release the shoulder and ribcage.

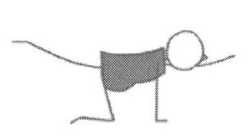

Extend right arm and left leg and hold for five breaths. Repeat other side.

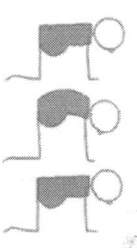

Come onto all fours with flat back. Inhale and curl the back upwards, look towards your bump. Exhale and back to flat back. Repeat x 10.

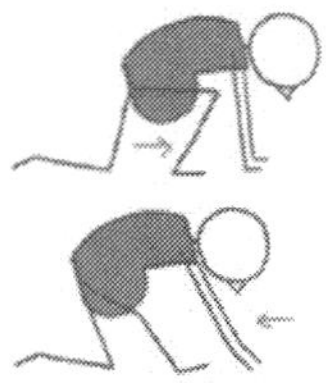

Move slowly from all fours to standing forward bend, as before.

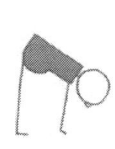

Exhale and bend forward as far as is comfortable. Bend knees if need to and take hands to knees, shins or floor. Use props as desired.

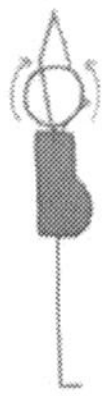

From forward fold, bend the knees and gently take the hands above the had in prayer on the inhale. Look up.

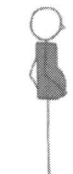

Exhale and come back to Tadasana (Mountain pose.)

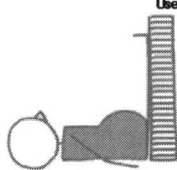

Allow yourself to relax in Savasana Corpse Cope or Vipritta Karani Legs Up the Wall Pose. Use cushions and blocks to prop up the hips. And rest.

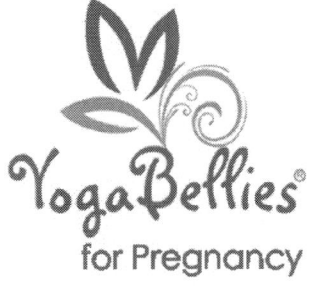

www.yogabellies.co.uk

YogaBellies® for Pregnancy

Mama Salutation

YogaBellies for Strength and Stamina in Pregnancy Sequence

This a strong, invigorating sequence perfect to wake you up in the morning, but also helps you build up strength and stamina for birthing. Depending on how well you feel, you can practice this routine throughout your pregnancy.

Hands Up
Always avoid taking your hands higher than the heart, if you suffer from high blood pressure or pre-eclampsia in pregnancy. As an alternative, take the hands to the hips or in front of your body in Prayer position.

Squatting
Squatting is brilliant in pregnancy, as it strengthens the length of the legs, tightens the buttocks. It helps us to build stamina and strength for birthing positions which require squatting or standing for long periods too. We wouldn't turn up a marathon without training, why do this at childbirth?
Use the support of the wall if you need to when squatting, especially when coming into a low squat. Don't take the feet as far apart as you normally would either. Do what feels comfortable and be sure not to over stretch. Wide leg squats should be avoided for people with pelvic girdle pain.

Pigeon Pose
Pigeon pose is possibly my favourite yoga posture of all time. It's fantastic for opening the hips and pelvic area and very therapeutic for Sciatica sufferers. Nudge yourself into it gently. If you can't stretch your back leg all the way out, come into a gentle variation called Mermaid Pose, where the front and back legs are bent more at the knee. Use a block under the buttocks for symmetry and comfort.

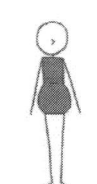

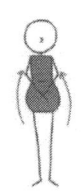

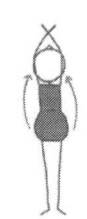

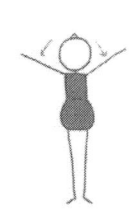

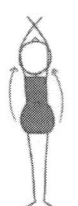

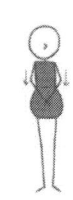

Stand in Mountain pose with feet hip width apart. Keep a gentle bend in the knees. Inhale as you bend elbows and raise arms above head, hands crossing body as you do so.

At the top look upwards, stretch the palms open and give thanks for the day ahead. Exhale as you lower the arms, continuing the circle

Continue the morning offering for 5-10 breaths. This beautiful stretch and grounding will wake you up.

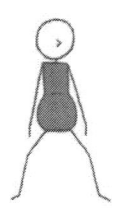

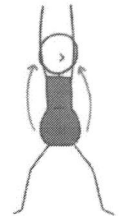

Stand with feet wider than hips, toes to 45 deg. Bend knees and exhale as come into Standing Goddess pose.

Inhale, straighten legs slightly and raise arms above head. Look up towards sky.

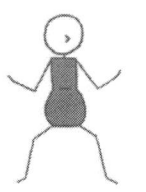

Stick out your tongue and make a loud "Ahhh" sound as bend knees and come back into Goddess pose. Repeat 5-10 times.

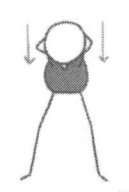

Keeping legs wide, take hands to hips and exhale as you bend forward from hips. Use wall for support if needed. Hold for 5 breaths.

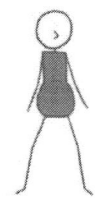

Come back into wide legged mountain pose and take a few breaths here.

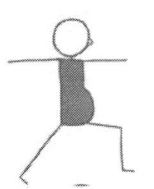

Take feet about 3 feet apart. R foot 90 degrees and back foot at 45. Bend R knee, raise arms and look towards R hand. Hold for 5 breaths and then rest R forearm on R thigh as bend forward. Raise L hand to sky and look up. Hold for 5 and repeat on L.

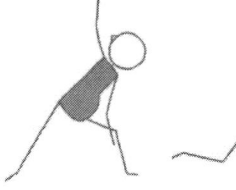

Slowly come to ground take R knee between hands and L leg extended behind.

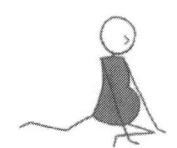

Straighten back, look forward and rest on fingertips. Look forward and take 5 breaths here. Come on to all fours and change sides.

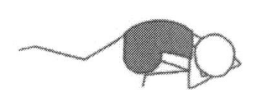

Bend forward, resting head on hands, birth ball or elbows to suit your bump. Rest here and relax.

Strength and Stamina Sequence

The Second Trimester and Crazy Cravings

The second trimester of pregnancy is commonly known as the most enjoyable time for mamas and it is often called pregnancy's 'honeymoon phase!' The worst is over, nausea has generally lessened or disappeared and you are starting to get your head around being pregnant.

This section contains more meal plans for guidance through the second trimester. It tells you is happening with mum and baby during at this time with some more Ayurvedic top tips. There are some YogaBellies for Pregnancy routines at the end too, suitable for every stage of pregnancy.

What's Happening with Mum and Baby in the Second Trimester?

This trimester is full of physical changes for your body and this is when you will really start to see a baby bump. You will notice your boobs getting bigger, and your belly growing as the baby makes itself at home in your body. You may notice stretch marks around your breasts and belly and it's common to have occasional leg cramps and dizziness too. This is all just your body adjusting to your pregnancy.

Fourth Month
In the fourth month, you may start to feel a 'heaviness' as your baby starts to grow and to become comfortable in your womb. All of baby's limbs and organs are now recognizable and the viscus of the heart, allows baby's consciousness to form. This is why mama should be placed on her lily pad during pregnancy, and given anything that she wants at this time.

Baby now has a neck, as well as joints in their arms and legs and hard bones beginning to develop. Baby is also now flexing and kicking, their skin begins to form, and they are now able to make facial expressions. Baby will be around 5 inches long at this time and will weigh less than 3 ounces.

Fifth month
In month five, baby is said to become conscious or a fully functioning mind (manah) and wakes up from its sleep of sub-conscious existence. Now baby is aware of everything that is going on outside of the womb and it's a great time to start bonding, if you haven't already.

Baby is now very active, kicking and moving around in your womb. Baby's sex organs are visible and a fine, hairy covering called lanugo that has developed. Baby's fat stores are beginning to develop and this is also when baby begins to hear. Your baby is now producing urine and they will even have teeny tiny eyebrows! Baby is about 6 inches long now and weighs almost 9 ounces.

Sixth Month
In the sixth month, baby's strength begins to increase and at the same time, you may notice that you begin to feel more tired. Feeling baby wriggle about is the most amazing feeling, and really helps you to connect with that little person growing inside of you. You may even experience an occasional kick or jab and baby will tend to start dancing when you attempt to meditate or go to sleep at night. Baby moving is a sign that they are healthy and well. Baby begins to straighten out at this point and a grayish-white, cheesy coating called vernix now covers baby's skin.

Along with the many physical changes for you and baby, you may also start to notice strange food cravings. This is because your tiny baby is growing bigger and needs lots of nutrition. During this trimester, you should gain around 4 pounds every month. Gaining weight is sign of a normal pregnancy, so don't panic when you start to get bigger.

Recommended Foods for the Second Trimester

Known to some as 'the golden trimester,' the second trimester is generally the easiest for mum to manage. Nausea and morning sickness have lessened and you will probably feel a lot more relaxed and energized. Gaining weight is an important and essential part of this trimester, but you should still be mobile and on the go.

Omega 3 fatty acids should be a vital part of your second trimester diet. They help to develop and nurture baby's brain and can be found in fish like salmon and mackerel.

During the second trimester, Calcium and Vitamin D are important nutrients that your body needs. These will help your baby to grow strong bones and some good Calcium rich foods include yoghurt, rice, milk, and cheese. Some great foods for you to stock up on Vitamin D include: fish, egg yolk, soy and fresh fruit smoothie. I've provided lots more examples in the 'foods you should be loving' section at the start.

As I mentioned before, foods rich in iron are very important throughout the entire pregnancy. Iron helps your body produce red blood cells and can be found in foods like porridge, chicken, lamb, dried fruits, spinach and green vegetables.

Meal Plans for the Second Trimester

Fourth Month

Meals Days	Breakfast	Lunch	Dinner
Monday	1 glass of Fresh fruit smoothie or milk. Porridge with milk with 1 tbsp. of sultanas and almonds.	1 Orange. Ciabatta bread with halloumi, sundried tomatoes and basil.	Chicken stir fry with zucchini noodles.
Tuesday	1 glass of fruit smoothie or milk. Wholegrain toast with sliced banana.	1 Pear. Broccoli and pea soup with a crusty wholegrain roll.	Creamy fish pie of haddock and salmon with Broccoli.
Wednesday	1 glass of Fresh fruit smoothie or milk. Greek yoghurt with Wheat cereal and fresh mixed berries.	A bowl of Chopped fruit. 1 Baked potato with coleslaw and tuna.	Carrot or Tridosha soup with whole grain bread.
Thursday	A cup of Herbal tea or milk. Fromage frais	1 Kiwi.	Pan-fried tuna steak. Sweet potato wedges

	mixed with 1 tbsp. of mixed berries. Toasted whole grain bagel with butter or ghee.	Smoked chicken and avocado salad.	and snap peas on the side.
Friday	1 glass of Yoghurt drink or milk. Porridge with milk with sliced bananas.	1 Apple. Fresh ham and cheese wholegrain sandwich.	Sweet apple lamb with couscous and spinach.
Saturday	Scrambled eggs with whole grain toast and butter or ghee. Fresh fruit smoothie or milk.	Toasted wholegrain bagel with butter or ghee and mashed banana	Vegetable curry with basmati rice.
Sunday	1 glass of Yoghurt drink or milk. Scotch pancakes with fresh blueberries.	Roast pork with roast parsnips, spring greens and potatoes.	Watercress and celery soup with a wholegrain roll.

Fifth Month

In month five, try to incorporate ghee (clarified butter) into your diet. It has loads of health benefits for pregnant women and is loaded with vitamins.

Meals Days	**Breakfast**	**Lunch**	**Dinner**
Monday	1 glass of Fresh fruit smoothie or milk. Porridge made in milk with 1 tbsp. of apple puree and a pinch of cinnamon.	1 Apple. Brown rice salad with mixed vegetables.	Chicken cassoulet with spinach.

Tuesday	1 fresh fruit smoothie A large bowl of Fromage Frais mixed with your choice of fresh fruits chopped and 1 tbsp. of almonds. Served with scotch pancakes.	Poached peaches. Masma Rasa (meaty soup)	Salmon with sweet potato wedges and pine nuts.
Wednesday	1 glass of Fresh fruit smoothie. Wheat cereal with milk and sliced bananas.	1 Orange. Salad of grapefruit, avocado, pomegranate, salad leaves, walnuts and feta cheese.	Pork and apple meatballs served with mashed potatoes and mange touts.
Thursday	1 cup of Herbal tea or milk. Porridge made in milk with 1 tbsp. of berry compote.	1 Kiwi. Baked potato and beans.	Grilled plaice fish with watercress and low-fat oven chips.
Friday	1 glass of Fresh fruit smoothie or milk. Wholegrain toast with smooth peanut butter.	1 Pear. Smoked chicken and avocado salad.	Beef and black bean casserole.
Saturday	1 cup of Herbal tea or milk. A large bowl of Greek yoghurt with chopped dried fruits of your choice, almonds and 1 tbsp. muesli.	Healthy BLT with grilled lean bacon, lettuce, thick slices of lean beef and tomato on granary bread.	Masma Rasa (meaty soup)

Sunday	1 Yoghurt drink. Scrambled eggs served on toasted bagel.	Roast chicken with Broccoli, potatoes and carrots. Baked apple with custard.	Tortilla with spicy tomato sauce, ham, spring onions and cheese.

Sixth Month

Try ghee boiled with sweet herbs like Liquorice, early in the morning on an empty stomach.

Meals / Days	Breakfast	Lunch	Dinner
Monday	1 glass of Fresh fruit smoothie. Porridge made in milk with 1 tbsp. of sultanas and almonds.	1 Pear. Baked potato with cheesy baked beans Pear	Chicken korma (spicy Indian chicken curry) with steamed rice.
Tuesday	1 Papaya smoothie Wholegrain toast with sliced bananas.	1 Orange. Cheddar cheese and tomato in a wholegrain roll	Pan-Fried salmon with pine nuts, potatoes and watercress.
Wednesday	1 glass of Fresh fruit smoothie. Wheat cereal with mixed berry compote and Greek yoghurt.	A small bunch of grapes Ciabatta bread with halloumi cheese, basil and sundried tomatoes.	Sweet apple lamb with mashed potatoes and broccoli.
Thursday	1 cup of Herbal tea. Fromage frais with 1 tbsp. of berry compote. Toasted bagel with peanut butter.	1 Apple. A bowl of chopped papaya. Salad of grapefruit, avocado, pomegranate,	Smoked mackerel fishcakes, served with spinach and cherry tomato salad.

		salad leaves, walnuts and feta cheese.	
Friday	1 Yoghurt drink. Porridge made in milk with sliced banana.	1 Kiwi. Smoked salmon, soft cheese on bagel. Poached pears.	Chili con carne served with rice.
Saturday	1 glass of Fresh fruit smoothie. Scrambled eggs served on toasted bagel	1 bowl of chopped papaya. Masma Rasa (meaty soup)	Homemade burgers with salad and fruity coleslaw.
Sunday	1 Yoghurt drink. Scotch pancakes with blueberries.	Fruit salad. Roast beef, potatoes, cauliflower and carrots with Cheese.	Watercress and celery soup with wholegrain roll.

YogaBellies in The Second Trimester

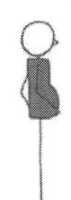

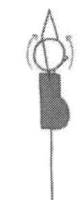

Stand in Mountain pose with feet hip width apart. Keep a gentle bend in the knees. Inhale as you bend elbows and raise arms above head, hands crossing body as you do so.

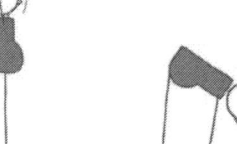

Exhale and bend forward as far as is comfortable. Bend knees if need to and take hands to knees, shins or floor. Use props as desired.

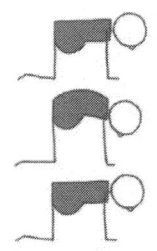

Come onto all fours with flat back. Inhale and curl the back upwards, look towards your bump. Exhale and back to flat back. Repeat x 10.

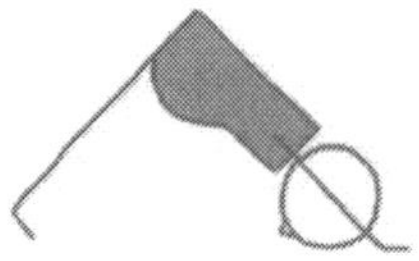

Pull up by the sit bones into Downward facing dog. Take the heels towards the mat but bend the knees if you have to. Press into hands.

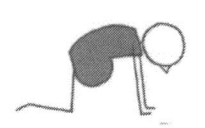

Come back to all fours and release the shoulder and ribcage.

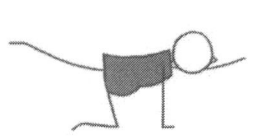

Extend right arm and left leg and hold for five breaths. Repeat other side.

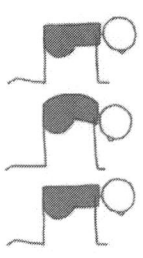

Come onto all fours with flat back. Inhale and curl the back upwards, look towards your bump. Exhale and back to flat back. Repeat x 10.

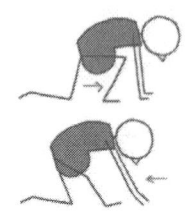

Move slowly from all fours to standing forward bend, as before.

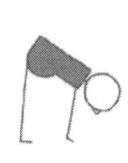

Exhale and bend forward as far as is comfortable. Bend knees if need to and take hands to knees, shins or floor. Use props as desired.

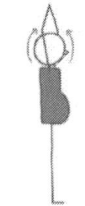

From forward fold, bend the knees and gently take the hands above the had in prayer on the inhale. Look up.

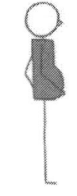

Exhale and come back to Tadasana (Mountain pose.)

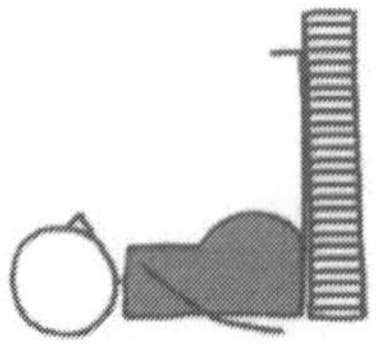

Allow yourself to relax in Savasana Corpse Cope or Viparitta Karani Legs Up the Wall Pose. Use cushions and blocks to prop up the hips. And rest.

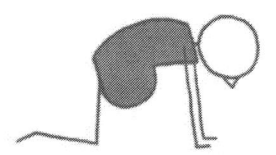

Come down onto all fours and release the shoulder and ribcage.

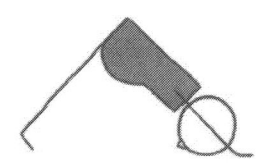

Pull up by the sit bones into Downward facing dog. Take the heels towards the mat but bend the knees if you have to. Take feet hip width or wider. Press into hands.

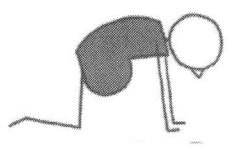

Come back to all fours and release the shoulder and ribcage.

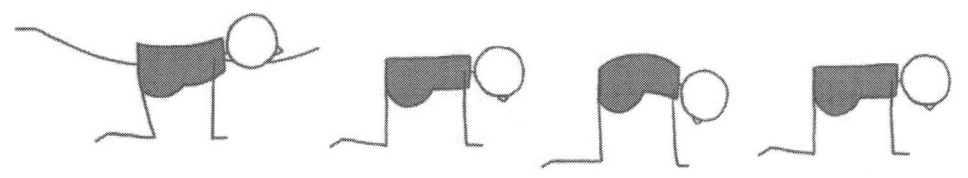

Extend right arm and left leg and hold for five breaths. Repeat other side.

Come onto all fours with flat back. Inhale and curl the back upwards, look towards your bump. Exhale and back to flat back. Repeat x 10.

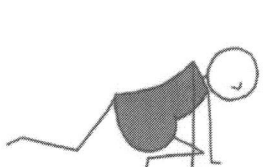

Gently move from all fours, bringing the R knee between the hands. Extend the L leg out behind as comfortable. Straighten back, take the shoulders back and look forward. Rest on fingertips. Lengthen the spine further by extended through top of the head and take 5 breaths here.

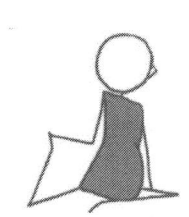

Take R hand to R foot. Take R foot towards buttocks. Hold for 5 breaths.

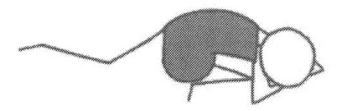

Lower the L leg back to the ground and take the forehead towards the mat, a block or birth ball for comfort. Rest here for 5 breaths and repeat on L.

Sciatica Routine

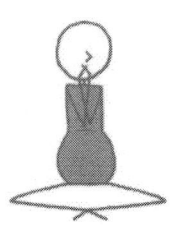

Come into Cobbler's Pose with soles of feet together. Take arms out front and cross R arm over L. Bring backs of hands together in prayer. Stretch hands up to sky and hold for 5.

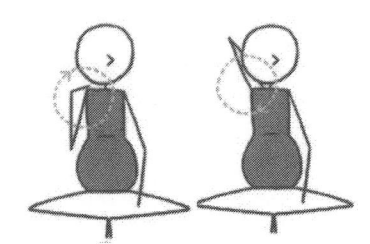

In Cobbler's Pose, Take R hand to R shoulder. Rotate elbow up and back in circular motion. Now repeat, bringing elbow forward. Continue as desired then repeat on L side.

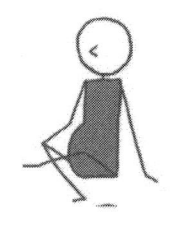

Come into Sukkashana (easy pose) or simple cross legged position.

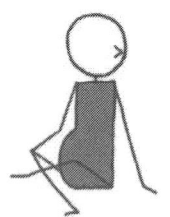

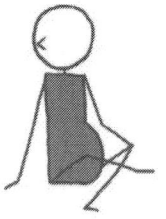

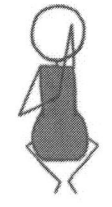

From Easy Pose, take the R hand to the R knee. Take the L hand behind the hips and place fingertips on the mat. Look over the L shoulder and enjoy an open rotation of the chest and heart. Keep spine straight and hold for 5 breaths and repeat on L side.

Come into Virasana (Hero Pose.) and sit on your heels. Take arms out front and cross R arm over L. Bring backs of hands together in prayer. Hold for 5. Repeat on L.

Take R arms above head. Take L hand behind back and ring hands together and clasp behind back Pull hands in opposing directions. Hold for 5. Repeat on L.

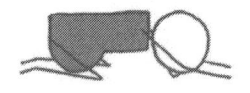

Come into Balasana (child's pose) keeping the knees wide to accommodate bump. Place hands on mat in front or head on block for comfort.

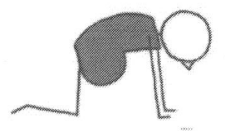

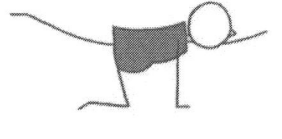

Come back to all fours and release the shoulders and ribcage.

Extend right arm and left leg and hold for five breaths. Repeat other side.

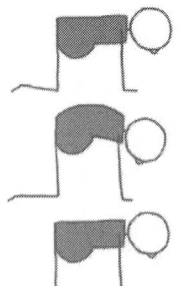

Come onto all fours with flat back. Inhale and curl the back upwards, look towards your bump. Exhale and back to flat back. Repeat x 10.

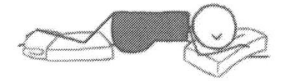

Come into side lying Savasana or Corpse Pose. Use blocks, cushions and blankets under the head and between knees and ankles to make you comfortable as appropriate. Rest.

Back Pain Sequence

The Third Trimester: Keep Going Mama!

The final hurdle! The third trimester is the most emotionally and physically challenging part of pregnancy. The position and size of your baby may make it more difficult for you to feel comfortable in any position at all, your ankles may be swollen (not that you can see them,) and you are just plain TIRED. In addition to this, you may be starting to stress about 'the big day.'

What's Happening with Mum and Baby in the Third Trimester?

Seventh Month
In month seven, you are starting to slow down. Your bump will now be big and heavy and it may be limiting your movement and activity. You will probably start to feel tired again around this time.

You may feel an itchy sensation on your chest or abdomen caused by baby's increased size. Gentle massage or friction can ease this.

All of baby's limbs are now developed and their brain is developing dramatically. Baby can suck now its thumb and show expressions responding to different tastes it experiences. Your baby's eyes can now open and close and its movements are stronger. You may feel baby's hiccups around this time. Baby now weighs 3 to 4 pounds.

Eight Month
In the eight month, Ayurveda states that energy moves back and forth between mother and baby which may cause you to experience fluctuating feelings of happiness and sadness, as they move back and forth. Ayurveda states that the constant transfer of energy, makes birthing in the eight-month higher risk.

Baby's head is now proportionate to the rest of their body and they should be moving at least 10 times every 2 hours. Movements won't be as strong now as baby has less room to move around. Baby is 16 to 19 inches long and weighs 6 pounds.

Ninth Month
Birthing normally takes place somewhere around mother's due date (2 weeks before and two weeks after is perfectly normal.)

The majority of baby's lanugo hair and vernix have now gone and their skin will be beautiful and soft. Baby is now shifting into to a head down position, ready for exit. Baby is around 20 inches and weighs around 8 pounds.

During the third trimester, your boobs will get even bigger (often leaking colostrum.) You may experience backaches, and a whole lot of heartburn. All fantastic fun! ☺ As the birth comes closer, you may also experience practice surges, known as Braxton Hicks contractions. These are not real contractions, but rather a warm-up for the real thing and a great opportunity to practice your YogaBellies Breathing techniques (see these later on.)

Through all of this, your emotions will be running high and you may still have fears and concerns about the pending childbirth. You may want to start spending time talking to your baby and planning ahead for the birth. Think about hiring a Doula (a professional birth companion,) to assist you and your partner on The Big Day. You should definitely consider attending positive antenatal classes and/or working with a Birth Mentor to help you prepare for birth using techniques such as hypnobirthing. Read positive birth books such as my book, Birth ROCKS or other inspiring birthing books such as Ina May's Guide to Childbirth or Hypnobirthing. You will be able to purchase all of these on Amazon.

Focus your energies on putting together a flexible birth plan and thinking about who you want to be your support person/people and where you would like to birth. Think about what you do and do not want for your birth. For example, where you want to birth, if you'd like to try for a water birth or if you would like to birth without drugs if possible. Staying calm is important. I cannot emphasize enough the support that you will gain from childbirth classes such as YogaBellies for Pregnancy or Birth ROCKS Hypnobirthing session with your partner. I am of course, entirely biased, but it's so true. I created these sessions to encourage support and community during a time when the rest of the world seems to want to terrify you.

Recommended Foods for the Third Trimester

The third trimester is the final stretch and soon you will be able to hold your gorgeous little person in your arms. This is a really important period to maintain your healthy diet and it benefits the last stages of growth for your baby.

In this trimester you can expect to gain at least another pound every week. Your baby will show some drastic growth in weight and size in this trimester too. Your bump may just suddenly 'pop out,' if you didn't have much of a bump before now.

Near the end of the third trimester you can expect to weight around 30 pounds more than you did before you became pregnant. Most of this weight is accounted for by the weight of your baby, but other reasons for weight gain are enlarged boobs, amniotic fluids, water retention and extra fat.

You may find you are no longer able to eat a full meal all at once, because your stomach is being pressed by your enlarged uterus. To avoid heartburn, it's best to divide your food into smaller meals throughout the day. If you are following the diet plan, split the meals into smaller portions and eat them a few hours apart to help aid digestion.

Vitamin K is important for birthing your child and breastfeeding. It helps the blood to clot and some great Vitamin K rich foods are things like: whole meal bread, green beans, watercress, melon and broccoli.

At this stage, it's likely that you will be less willing or able to move around less and you will be more prone to indigestion. Try to really cut back on the coffee and spicy food (although reintroducing the curries nearer the Big Day, can help move things along.)

You need to make sure that you are eating food that will boost your energy and provide at lots of Calcium every day too. Energy boosting foods could include things like baked beans, fruits, cheese peanut butter, etc.

Snacking throughout the day can be great at this stage too, as you will need an extra 200 calories every day during this trimester. Nausea may also have started to return towards the end of the third trimester, so healthy snacks can help keep any sickie feelings at bay too.

Meal Plans for The Third Trimester

You will need more energy in the third trimester as your baby continues to grow and deplete your energy stores. Baby's fat stores continue to accumulate during this trimester and their organ function continues to improve.

Seventh Month

Tops tips for the seventh month of pregnancy...

- In month seven, continue to follow your routine from month six.
- Eat food in smaller quantities and don't add extra fat or salt to your food.
- From time to time, take a bite of sweet something with little ghee or oil so that it is easy to digest.
- Try to avoid drinking water immediately after a meal also.

Meals Days	Breakfast	Morning Snack	Lunch	Evening Snack	Dinner
Monday	1 glass apple juice or milk. Porridge made in milk with 1 tbsp. apple puree and a pinch of cinnamon.	1 small roll with butter or ghee,	1 satsuma. Couscous and egg salad with currants and pine nuts.	Hummus with carrot sticks.	Smoked mackerel with baby spinach.
Tuesday	A fresh fruit smoothie Fromage frais mixed with fresh fruits and 1 tbsp. flaked almonds. Served with	Masma Rasa (meaty soup)	A Small bunch of grapes Roast beef in a wholegrain baguette with rocket.	1 thick slice of banana bread.	Creamy curry of chickpeas.

	Scotch pancakes.				
Wednesday	1 glass apple juice or milk Wheat cereal, milk and sliced bananas.	Yoghurt with blueberries and melon.	A bowl of chopped melon. Beetroot soup.	Rye crackers with sardine paste.	Chicken and basmati rice risotto.
Thursday	1 cup of herbal tea or milk. Porridge made in milk with 1 tbsp. of fresh berries.	1 thick slice of a whole grain toast with butter or ghee.	1 sliced mango Pita with lamb's lettuce, Gruyere and grapes.	Cup of Masma Rasa (meaty soup)	Creamy fish pie of haddock and salmon with green beans.
Friday	A yoghurt drink or milk Wholegrain toast with butter or ghee.	2 handfuls of dried fruits, including walnuts.	1 apple Salad of watercress and salmon.	Fruity flapjacks.	Lamb chops with mange tout and sweet potato wedges.
Saturday	1 glass orange juice or milk. Greek yoghurt with a tbsp. of dried fruits and muesli.	A rice pot.	1 Pear Toasted whole grain ham and cheese sandwich.	Whole meal toast topped with butter or ghee.	Lean beef lasagna and leafy green salad on the side.
Sunday	A yoghurt drink or milk.	1 fresh fruit smoothie	Roasted lamb, green	Cheese on wholegrain toast.	A quiche of cheese

| | Scrambled eggs on a toasted bagel. | | beans and carrots with rice pudding. | | and spinach. |

Eighth Month

In month eight, try eating rice prepared with milk in semi-solid or liquid form with ghee. Sweet gruel prepared in milk also proves beneficial if eaten in this month. You can have gruel made of rice, sooji or wheat vermicelli.

Meals Days	Breakfast	Morning Snack	Lunch	Evening Snack	Dinner
Monday	Apple juice or milk. Porridge made in milk with 1 tbsp. of sultanas. 1 slice whole meal toast with butter or ghee.	Melon and blueberries with yoghurt.	1 kiwi. Beetroot soup, a crusty wholegrain roll on the side.	1 orange	Creamy curry of chickpeas with basmati rice.
Tuesday	1 fruit smoothie or milk. Whole meal toast with butter and sliced bananas.	Hummus with pita bread.	1 orange. Couscous and egg salad, with currants and pine nuts.	Rye crackers spread with cheddar cheese.	Creamy fish pie of salmon, haddock, and peas.
Wednesday	Orange juice or milk. Wheat cereal, mixed berries and Greek	Oat, orange and cranberry cookie.	1 bowl of chopped Melon. Tuna salad wholegrain wrap or salad.	Sweet gruel prepared in milk	Masma rasa (meaty soup)

	yoghurt with 2 Scotch pancakes.				
Thursday	1 cup herbal tea or milk. Fromage frais, 1 tbsp. of chopped Berries.	Whole meal bread with butter or ghee.	1 apple. Smoked salmon bagel.	Hummus with pita bread.	Chicken with tomato and stir fry zucchini noodles.
Friday	1 yoghurt drink or milk. Porridge in milk with sliced bananas.	Sweet gruel prepared in milk	1 pear. Baked potato with lean beef chili.	1 slice of gingerbread.	Sweet apple lamb, mashed potatoes, carrots and green beans.
Saturday	Orange juice. Scrambled eggs and whole meal toast.	Sweet gruel prepared in milk	Cheese, broccoli and cauliflower pasta. Fruit salad.	2 slices of whole meal toast with ghee or butter	Grilled beef steak and broccoli with butternut squash and sweet potato mash.
Sunday	1 yoghurt drink or milk. Scotch pancakes	1 mixed fruit smoothie.	Roast chicken, potatoes with carrots and	Cheese on wholegrain toast.	A quiche of cheese and spinach with salad.

| | with blueberries. | | mange tout. Poached pears. | | |

Ninth Month

Meals / Days	Breakfast	Morning Snack	Lunch	Evening Snack	Dinner
Monday	Apple juice or milk. Porridge made in milk with 1 tbsp. of sultanas. 1 whole meal toast with butter or ghee.	Melon and blueberries with yoghurt.	Beetroot soup with a crusty wholegrain roll with butter. Kiwi fruit	1 orange.	Creamy curry of chickpeas with rice.
Tuesday	1 fresh fruit smoothie. Whole meal toast with butter and sliced bananas.	Hummus with pita bread.	1 orange. Couscous and egg salad, with currants and pine nuts.	Rye crackers spread with cheese.	Creamy fish pie of salmon, haddock, and peas.
Wednesday	Orange juice or milk. Wheat cereal, mixed berries and Greek yoghurt with 2 Scotch pancakes.	Oat, orange and cranberry cookie.	1 bowl of chopped Melon. Tuna salad wrap.	Sweet gruel prepared in milk	Penne with spinach, and tomato based sauce.
Thursday	1 cup herbal tea or milk.	Whole meal bread with	1 apple. Sardines on toast.	Hummus with pita bread.	Lamb and veg casserole.

	Fromage frais, 1 tbsp. of fresh berries.	butter and rice with vegetables			
Friday	1 Yoghurt drink or milk. Porridge in milk with sliced bananas.	Sweet gruel prepared in milk	1 pear. Baked potato with lean beef chili.	1 slice of gingerbread	Grilled pork chops with mashed potatoes, carrots and green beans.
Saturday	Orange juice. Scrambled eggs and a whole meal toast.	1 fresh fruit smoothie Apple and bran muffin.	Cheese and cauliflower pasta. Fruit salad.	Whole meal toast with organic baked beans.	Grilled beef steak and broccoli with butternut squash and sweet potato mash.
Sunday	1 yoghurt drink. Scotch pancakes with blueberries.	2 handfuls of dried fruits.	Roasted chicken, potatoes and mange tout. Poached pear crunch.	Cheese on wholegrain toast.	A quiche of cheese and spinach with salad.

YogaBellies in the Third Trimester

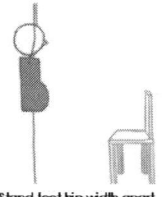

Stand feet hip width apart and raise arms above head in prayer. Stretch up with gentle back bend. Look up.

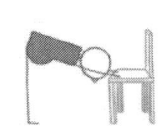

Exhale and bend forward, hold onto edge of stable seat. Allow bump to hang and relax. Take 5 breaths here.

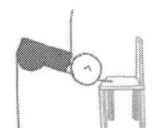

Inhale and raise R hand to sky. Look towards hand. Enjoy the rotation. Hold for five breaths and repeat on L side.

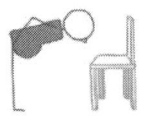

Take the hands to the hips, gently bend knees and inhale as you come back to standing.

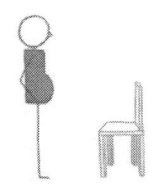

Take five breaths in Tadasana (mountain pose.)

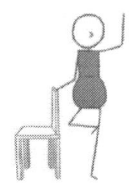

Holding back of chair, take right foot to shin or thigh. Take L arm to hip or above head. Hold for five and repeat on L side.

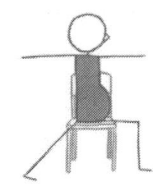

Use chair as support for warrior. R foot 90 degrees and L foot at 45. Look at R hand. Hold for 5 and repeat on L.

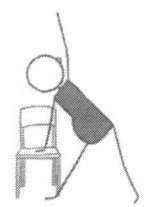

Feet about foot apart. R foot 90 deg and L at 45. Rest right hand to chair, extend L hand to sky. Look at L hand. 5 breaths and repeat on L.

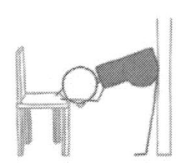

Stand against wall and bend forward, taking hands to chair. Relax and soften knees for 5 breaths.

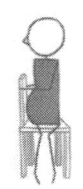

Sit sideways on chair holding back. Twist chest to right, hold for 5 breaths and repeat on L.

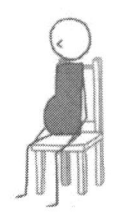

Sit back against chair back with feet on ground. Take 5 breaths here.

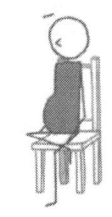

Take R foot to L knee. Extend R knee towards ground for 5 breaths. Repeat on L side.

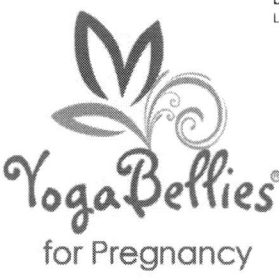

Chair Yoga Sequence

A great sequence when you just need a little extra support. Perfect for the third trimester when baby is becoming heavy but you still want to stretch and strengthen. This sequence will keep you strong and grounded.

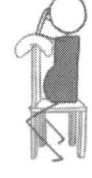

Sit facing chair back. Place cushion or support on back. Rest elbows or forehead on chair back and relax here as long as you need to. Bring attention to the breath and rest...

YogaBellies for Pregnancy

www.yogabellies.co.uk

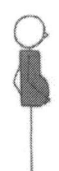

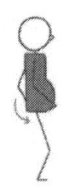

Stand in Mountain pose with feet hip width apart. Keep a gentle bend in the knees. Inhale as you tilt the pelvis forward and exhale as you come back. Take the hands to the hips as you do so.

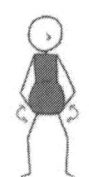

Keeping hands on hips, bend the knees and circle the hips in a clockwise direction. Rotate in the opposite direction until hips release.

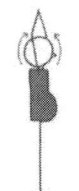

Inhale and raise arms above head in prayer. Stretch upwards and then to R for 5 breaths and then L for 5.

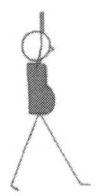

Take feet about 3 feet apart, R foot 90 degrees and back foot at 45. Raise arms in prayer and look forwards.

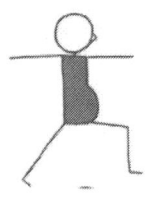

Bend R knee and come into Warrior 2. Raise arms parallel to ground and look over R hand. Hold for 5 and repeat on L.

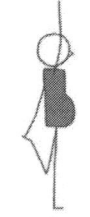

Stand close to wall or hold and take R foot to buttocks. Take forehead to wall and raise R foot to sky as comfortable. Repeat on L.

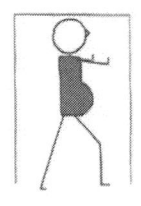

Press hands against wall and push into R foot. Take L foot behind and push into heel and hands stretching calves. Repeat on other side.

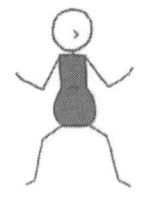

Come back into Goddess pose and take a few breaths here.

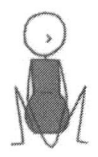

With back against wall slide down into seated squat pose. Take 10 breaths here.

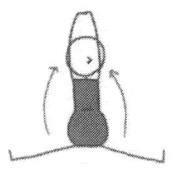

Stretch the legs out as far as is comfortable and point toes up. Clasp hands and raise over head and stretch up.

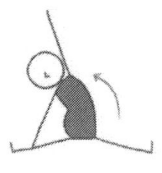

Take R hand to thigh and left hand up and over to the R. Hold for 5 breaths and repeat on other side.

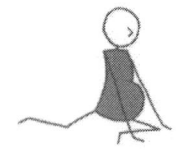

Straighten back, look forward and rest on fingertips. Look forward and take 5 breaths here. Come to all fours and change sides.

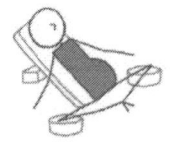

Use props, blankets and cushions to make yourself comfortable in reclined cobblers pose. Bring soles of feet together and allow the knees to open. Rest.

Hips and Pelvis Sequence

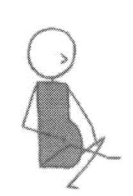

Sit in simple cross legged position. Use cushions under the knees or sit against wall for comfort if required.

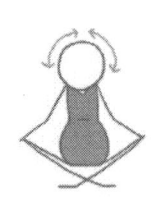

Close your eyes and circle the head around the neck and the shoulders, to the left, to the right and all the way round.

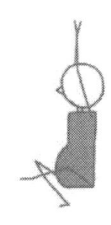

Bring palms together in prayer and raise and lower hands above head x 10. Inhale UP Exhale DOWN.

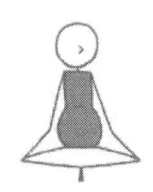

Come into Cobblers Pose with soles of the feet together and hands on knees.

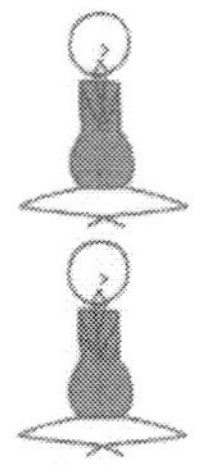

In Cobbler or Cross Leg, cross arms over each other at elbows and bring back of hands together. Raise arms and look up to sky.

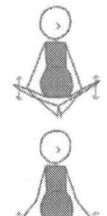

Holding knees or feet, flex the knees up and down, releasing the hips.

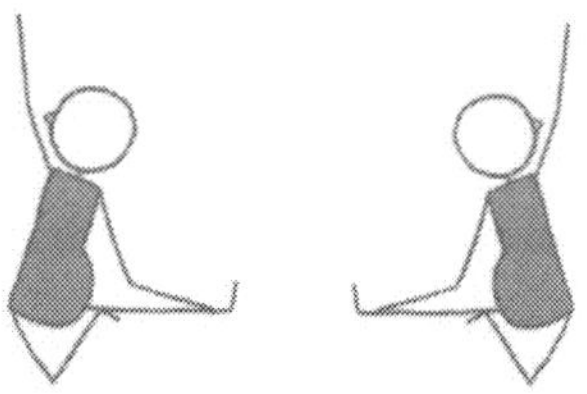

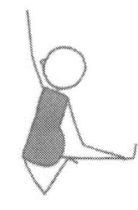

Come into Revolved Head to Knee Pose by taking the right heel to the groin and extending the left leg out. Grab left toe/shin and raise right arm up and over head and . Hold for five. Repeat on opposite side.

Come into Child's Pose. Take head to mat or block, spread knees to accommodate bump and rest.

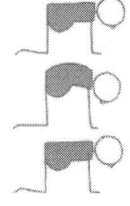

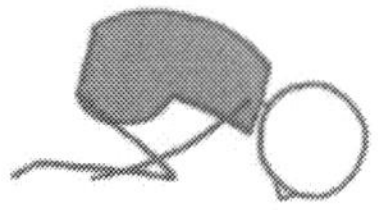

Come onto all fours with flat back. Inhale and curl the back upwards, look towards your bump. Exhale and back to flat back. Repeat x 10.

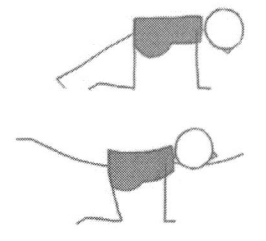

Extend right foot behind, come onto toes and extend heel to ground. Hold for 5 and repeat other side.

Extend right arm and left leg and hold for five breaths. Repeat other side.

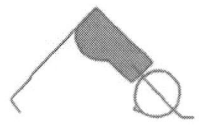

From all fours, push into the heels and come into Downward facing dog. Push into the hands and lengthen spine all way to buttocks. Take weight into the heels and bend knees if you have to.

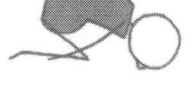

Come into Child's Pose. Take head to mat or block, spread knees to accommodate bump and rest.

Seated Sequence

A great sequence suitable for all stages of pregnancy.

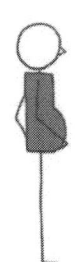

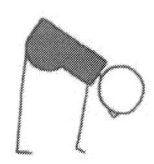

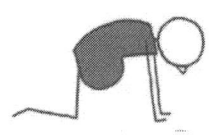

Stand in Mountain pose with feet hip width apart. Keep a gentle bend in the knees. Inhale as you bend elbows and raise arms above head, hands crossing the body as you do so.

Exhale and bend forward as far as is comfortable. Bend knees if need to and take hands to knees, shins or floor. Use props as desired.

Come back to all fours and release the shoulders and ribcage.

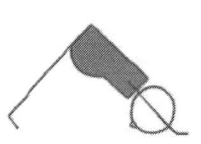

Pull up by the sit bones into Downward facing dog. Take the heels towards the mat but bend the knees if you have to. Press into hands and lengthen spine.

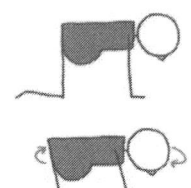

Come back onto all fours. Look over the R shoulder towards the R hip. Bring R hip towards the head. Hold for 5 breaths and repeat on L side. Do 3 rounds.

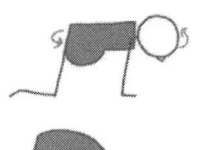

From kneeling, place forehead on mat, and keep buttocks high. Sway hips from side to side as comfortable.

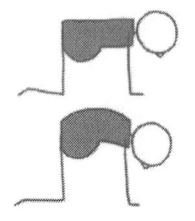

Come onto all fours with flat back. Inhale and curl the back upwards, look towards your bump. Exhale and back to flat back. Repeat x 10.

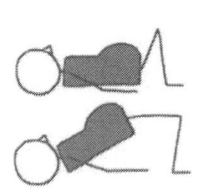

Come onto your back (if comfortable to do so.) Bend the knees, feet on floor and press back of forearms and palms into mat. Raise the hips slowly towards the sky and hold for 5 breaths. Lower and repeat.

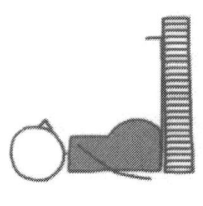

Allow yourself to relax in Savasana Corpse Cope or Viparitta Karani Legs Up the Wall Pose. Use cushions and blocks to prop up the hips. And rest.

Breech Baby Sequence

Nutrition in Pregnancy: QUICK REMINDERS

- Look after yourself and take time to rest and recuperate when you need it;
- Eat well throughout pregnancy;
- Try to avoid fast-food, ice-cream, additives and any nasties;
- Try to include some Ayurvedic remedies and supplements into your pregnancy diet plan;
- But don't be too hard on yourself if you slip sometimes…
- Drink LOTS of water, at least 8 glasses per day;
- Always plan your shopping list to avoid cheating!
- If you can't finish a whole meal, split them into 'mini meals' and snack throughout the day;
- Always try to eat fresh, whole, organic foods during pregnancy where possible;
- Remember that every lovely thing you eat goes into creating and growing your baby!

The Fourth Trimester and Post-Partum Mama

Ayurveda for Postpartum Mama

After the birth, you will have a lot recuperating to do. Your body, mind and hormones have been working hard and there is a high chance that you will be completely exhausted.

Six Weeks Just for Mama

Getting to know your new baby, while trying to adapt to the demands of motherhood, can be a difficult balancing act. In Ayurveda, a strong emphasis is placed on the 42 days, or 6 weeks after childbirth. This is one of the most significant periods of a woman's life, and one which will impact greatly on your health in years to come.

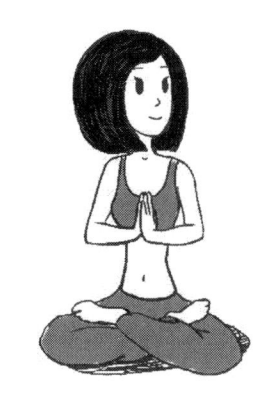

In western culture, it is very easy to jump back into workouts and working, and fall prey to the hamster-wheel of running until we burn out. A new mum should take every opportunity to rest while baby is resting. Mum should rely heavily on her partner (if possible,) as well as other family members and the support of friends.

Cleaning, cooking and other household duties should be delegated in the last few weeks of pregnancy, so that you can relax when you need to. If you don't get the rest that you need, then taking care of baby can become overwhelming, and you may feel fatigued and even depressed.

Soothing Post-Partum Mama

In a matter of hours after giving birth, mum will lose around 15 pounds of weight directly from the abdomen, known as the 'seat of Vata.' 'Vata' is comprised of air and space, which is exactly what is left in your body after baby is born. In addition to this, the major changes that your body has undergone over the last 9 months have all come to a head, with a most likely exhausting, birthing experience. This is why in Ayurveda; we would give special attention to decreasing Vata at this time.

Simple Ways to care for Post-Partum Mama

- Mum should be kept warm and safe, in a familiar environment;
- Soothing massage using warm oils, can help to moisturize and soothe mother in the post-partum period (see Abhyanga ;)
- Creating a routine for feeding, bathing and sleeping, as much as is possible, will help you remain positive and become used to motherhood.
- Taking time to be still and to rest will help to replenish and nourish mama.

Postpartum Abhyanga

In Ayurvedic traditions, it is recommended that postpartum 'Abhyanga' is performed daily, by a skilled Ayurvedic Postpartum Therapist. The practitioner comes to your home, so that you can have baby nearby in case you need to nurse at any point during the treatment. A lot of oil is applied, more than a typical Abhyanga, as it is very hydrating and has a vata-reducing quality. Herbalized oils can help to soothe soreness and restore energy and vitality.

Aggravated Vata is soothed dramatically by massage, so it's important to realize how vital massage is to mum's postpartum healing. It can be expensive and slightly unrealistic to have massages daily for the entire 6 weeks, so any soothing massage by friends or family will be just as good. Massage should be followed by warm bath and deep rest.

As a new mum, we feel guilty doing anything at all for ourselves, and I know that I ran around looking like a crazy person, with wild hair and pretty unkempt. We are completely focused on the care of our new baby and it's so easy to forget that your care and rest is just as important. Don't feel selfish looking after yourself. If you are not rested and well, you won't be able to give your all to baby.

Ayurvedic Dietary Guidelines for Post-Partum

Agni (your digestive fire,) is at its lowest in the period directly following childbirth. This is because so much energy and focus in your body, was on making sure that baby came safely and smoothly into the world.

'Kindling the digestive fire' is very important in the post-partum period. Begin to slowly add foods back into your diet. It is very important to continue to eat a Vata-balancing diet during the postpartum period, for you and baby's ongoing wellbeing.

Some Signs of a Vata Excess:

- Gas (this appears in an infant as colic),
- Poor or disrupted sleeping patterns,
- Chronic tiredness,
- Constipation.

In the days following birth, food for post-partum mama should be soupy, warm, sweet and easily-digestible. Foods like ghee, sweet grains, avocado, soaked nuts, warm cereals, sweet vegetables, fruits and milk are most soothing at this time.

It is important to avoid vegetables like Brussel sprouts, garlic, broccoli, peppers, greens, potatoes, fermented cheeses, cauliflower, onions, chilies, yeasted breads, corn, and dry foods such as crackers. These foods are said to increase the air element in the body.

If you have time off work before baby arrives, you can prepare meals and freeze them for defrosting after the birth. Ideally food will be prepared freshly, to ensure that it is Sattvic, but let's be practical.

Mama Mocktails

As mentioned, Agni decreases dramatically after a woman gives birth and emphasis should be placed on 'rekindling that fire.' I've included a couple of recipes for you to put together at home, to help do just that.

Mama Mojito: My Ayurvedic Energy Drink for New Mamas

Here is a great recipe for a very beneficial Ojas-increasing energy drink that is just perfect for breastfeeding mothers:
10 blanched almonds, skinned,
1 cup of boiled milk,
3 dates,
A pinch of cardamom,
A thread of saffron, blended.

Mummy Sunrise: Rekindle the Fire

One of the best ways to improve Agni, is to blend yourself together a 'Mummy Sunrise.' Mix together water with:
Cumin
Coriander
Fennel

Pop it in a martini glass and drink it first thing in the morning: what an awesome way to perk up your morning! Warming spices in general, will aid your digestion and help to make your 'Agni' stronger.

Ayurveda provides so much brilliant and highly applicable knowledge and support for mums throughout the childbearing years. It can be difficult just to find your toothbrush in the morning immediately post-partum, so approach this Ayurvedic advice with an accepting mind-set. These ancient principles can give you much needed guidance and comfort in the unknown terrain that is post-partum, but if you can't manage to do it all like it says in the book, that's okay too.

Rocking Your Beautiful New Body

Once the birth is over, your baby is happily in your arms, and you're heading back home, you suddenly realize that the big changes are just about to start.

Over the next few months, your entire life will change in more ways than you could ever imagine. This can be pretty daunting, and it will take time for you to get used to being a new mum or the mum of more than one. This tiny new addition to the family is going to take some getting used to.

Aside from all the changes to your day to day life, you will probably begin thinking about how your body looks post-birth, and wonder if it will ever look the same again. During pregnancy, everyone gains weight and that's natural and healthy. Now that baby is here, you'll probably want to go back to being able to fit into that favourite pair of jeans. Not so fast mama!

You will quickly realize that this is not going to happen overnight. What you may not have accounted for, is the fact that with a new-born in your life, it isn't that easy to find the time or energy to get back into shape quickly.

Don't become disheartened. In fact, jumping straight back into your pre-pregnancy workout is actually the worst thing you can do. Although it might not be entirely as easy as you expected, you can definitely get back into terrific shape. The most important thing is to focus on three key areas or as I like to call them: The BAP's (Your Back, Abs and Pelvic floor.) We'll take more about this later.

Here's a newsflash:

Your body will NEVER look the same again.

This is not necessarily a bad thing and it doesn't mean that you will forever have a baby paunch. It does mean that your hips, pelvis and butt will have changed shape. It doesn't mean you can't work them back into a good shape, but ultimately the actual shape, will have changed. In fact, you may find that you prefer your new shape, with broader hips and more rounded breasts. Especially if you now find yourself a seasoned yogi! Before you jump into trying to shed the pounds, let's look at how your baby weight is made up.

Pregnancy Weight Gain and Acceptance

We all know that it is normal to gain some weight during pregnancy. After all, you are carrying a whole entire new life within your body, and so that's bound to weigh you down.

Generally speaking, the weight that you do gain can actually be broken down into a number of elements that comprise the total weight, and these are:

Baby – 8 pounds

Maternal fat and nutrient stores – 7 pounds

Uterus – 2 pounds

Placenta – 2 pounds

Amniotic fluid – 2 pounds

Maternal blood – 4 pounds

Maternal breast tissue – 2 pounds

Fluid in maternal tissue – 4 pounds

This equates to around 31 pounds. Bear in mind though that this is not an exact figure, but for someone who was at a healthy weight before pregnancy, the average ideal weight gain during pregnancy is around 25 to 37 pounds.

On the other hand, if you were underweight before pregnancy, you would probably gain 28 to 40 pounds, whereas if you were overweight, it would be normal to gain 15 to 25 pounds. Remember to consider your pre-pregnancy weight and size when looking at these figures.

If you're asking yourself why the difference in weight gain exists, then simply think of it like this. In addition to all of the baby-related weight gain factors listed, the final factor is pregnancy weight and nutrient stores. These stores are essentially stored up energy that you and your baby will need for growth and repair, and they're just like any other energy stores. Soon you'll see how this links in with losing weight, but for now, just keep it in mind.

Suffice to say, if you were overweight initially, you'll need less energy stores, whereas if you were underweight, you'll need more.

Another thing to keep in mind is the fact that, you really aren't gaining that much weight, outside of your pregnancy. Most of what you do gain can, and will, be lost after birth. All that remains are mainly those energy stores that we just talked about.

This is the ideal situation but the truth is that many of us will actually gain more weight during pregnancy than we 'ideally' should. Those Big Mac's and Dairy Milk's are sometimes too much to resist. Even if you do indulge, you can still shed those extra pounds' post-partum by approaching it in the right way.

Focus on Positive Movement, Not Weight Loss

Lots of women jump into sit ups (Just don't!) and HITT training and weights, when baby is just a few days old. Please don't do this! Nothing could be more detrimental to your health, wellbeing, recovery and sanity.

Making sure that you are moving every day, taking baby out to the park or the shops, taking even five minutes for a gentle yoga practice or meditation, all of these things are so much more valuable in the immediate post-natal period, than pounding the treadmill. Chillax and spend quality time with your baby, the rest will come in time.

Post Natal Yoga is the perfect way to begin to gently move again, and will naturally guide your body back to (almost) its former self. Also, if you find a YogaBellies for Mum & Baby class, you can incorporate baby into your yoga practice, and you both benefit. What could be more rewarding than that?

Post Natal Yoga: With and Without Baby

You Can Practice Yoga with Your Baby

I often say to mummies when they come along to mum and baby yoga, that practicing yoga with your child is the most yogic thing you will ever do. Suddenly, you realize it's not all about you anymore. Mums come along, yoga mat in one arm, baby in the other looking forward to lovely rewarding stretch and a nice deep relaxation at the end – maybe even a much needed afternoon snooze. But as anyone who has tried yoga with baby will know, it doesn't always work like that ☺

Yoga with baby takes patience and acceptance that you may not manage the physical yoga practice you want to do. Baby could be feeding or sleeping or crying. The most important lesson we learn from yoga here, is that it's all okay. It IS possible to relax with baby; it just may not look the way it used to.

Why would I do Yoga with my Baby?

Post-natal yoga has been proven to help minimize post-natal depression, helping you to adjust to life as a parent and helping you communicate better with your new baby. As well as emotional and physical improvements, you will be able to focus on rebuilding your weakened pelvic floor; strengthen your abdominal muscles and even help alleviate any back or neck pain.

For babies, yoga can help with common complaints such as digestion and colic; help to strengthen their tiny limbs, improve sleep patterns and enhance their ability to interact with mum and other people.

What's the Difference between Post-Natal Yoga for Mum and Baby Yoga?

Post-natal and baby yoga are two distinct areas of yoga that are often muddled up or mis-sold. They actually work best when practiced together. As you will very quickly come to realize, every activity from now on will involve baby, and what better an opportunity to embrace this than in your yoga class? Post-natal, baby yoga and mum and baby yoga classes are now widely available across the UK, although yoga with baby is no new thing.

Baby yoga and massage have been practiced for thousands of years in India and even today in India, yoga and massage with baby are as important as a daily bath.

The benefits of post-natal yoga (yoga for mummy post-birth) have been widely recognized in the past twenty years in the western world as the practice of yoga has been adapted to work with the female body. Just as during pregnancy, you have to be kind to your body and take things at a gentler pace. You need to gradually build up back to your normal level of activity post-partum.

When Can I Start Post-Natal Yoga?

In YogaBellies for Mum and Baby classes, I always advise mums to wait until 6-8 weeks after the birth for a normal birth or at least 10 weeks for a C-section. The most important thing is that you listen to your body and are guided by how you personally feel post-partum. You should not exercise the pelvic floor muscles until there is no pain in that area: bruised muscles should never be exercised and the same applies to your pelvic floor.

Many post-natal exercise classes today advise mums go directly into intense physical exercise regimes in order to regain their pre-pregnancy shape and lose their mummy bump. This really is the worst possible thing you can do.

Many mothers neglect the rebuilding of the pelvic floor, and return to sit ups and strenuous work out regimes as soon as possible. This results in a weakened pelvic floor, abdominal muscles which have not recovered (if you jump into sit ups you could end up with a 'six pack' and protruding lower abdominals) and very often on-going lower back pain also. By strengthening the pelvic floor and lower abdominals, we also help strengthen the lower back and integrity of the spinal cord.

My Baby Can Do Yoga?

'Baby yoga' is when mum gently manipulates baby's little body in yoga postures or 'asana.' Now this sounds scary, but it's actually a very lovely and gentle practice. We don't hold babies upside down or swing them about: that is NOT baby yoga, I believe that is called child abuse ☺

Thousands of years ago, yoga masters based adult yoga postures of the movements that new babies make naturally as they begin to move about (think about Happy Baby Pose: where the yoga lies on their back and grabs their toes – something babies do a lot!)

New babies today are often physically restricted in ways they were not in the past. Babies spend a lot of time in buggies, cots and car seats or bouncing chairs or swings. Babies can actually become stressed and stiff just like adults. One of the reasons we practice baby yoga is to help strengthen baby's body and encourage flexibility. The best thing is that by practicing yoga with baby, and demonstrating deep breathing and relaxation with baby, we are actually teaching them the principals of relaxation at an early age.

Baby yoga sessions also help stimulate baby's brain development using a range of movement – making them aware of things like their toes (think about how excited a baby is when they realize they have toes! It's big news.)

Baby yoga also teaches your baby to self soothe and how to become calm and still. At the end of a mum and baby yoga session, you will often find that baby is happily exhausted, relaxed and fast asleep: always a bonus if you are heading home to attempt making a family meal.

What does a Mum and Baby Yoga Session Involve?

There are many variations to the structure of a 'post-natal' or 'baby yoga' class. It is important that you understand the differences in these classes, to make sure that you get as much as possible from the sessions. A post-natal yoga class will focus on post-partum mother. Your baby is usually left in the buggy or placed to one side, while the focus of the session is concentrated on you.

A baby yoga class focuses on yoga for baby, aiming to help baby grow strong and healthy, often an extension of a baby massage class. This is a not a post-partum yoga class and the focus in on your baby rather than you.
The best post-partum yoga classes, involve a mixture of yoga for mum AND baby. Ideally the class should involve post-natal yoga postures helping to strengthen mothers mind and body as well as incorporating your baby into your yoga practice, including asanas to help their little bodies too.

Mum and baby yoga classes of this format are superior in that they encourage you to bond with your baby and help you understand that your baby must now be incorporated into every aspect of your life. I have often said that yoga with baby is the most yogic thing you will ever do as you quickly come to realize that it's not all about you anymore.

From time to time, baby will cry or want to feed during the session and so you may not have the active session you hoped for. Yoga breathing techniques and relaxation are also taught in class which can help you relax with baby (yes it is possible) and to embrace this new responsibility.

What should I look for in a Mum and Baby Yoga Teacher?

It is vitally important that your teacher has had specific training in these areas. Ideally, those teaching post-natal yoga have completed a 200-hour yoga teacher training qualification accredited by organizations such as the IYN (Independent Yoga Network) or Yoga Alliance in the first instance. The teachers should then have had subsequent training in the areas of post-natal yoga and/or baby yoga depending on what they teach. You should always make sure their teacher is associated with and supported by a reputable organization.

They must be able to work safely and sensitively with you and your baby at this special time.

Some Signs that You're Not Ready to Practice Yet

Whether you like it or not, after birth, you will be in a somewhat fragile condition and need time to rest and recover. Even if you were in great shape prior to pregnancy, even if you had a dream birth, the changes that your body has gone through over the last nine months will definitely have had a huge impact and you need time to recover.

After childbirth, those changes are going to continue to have an effect for a few weeks, or even months. Bearing this in mind, you will need to limit any strenuous activity. Pushing yourself as hard as you can is definitely off the table, and you can't train as if you're trying to compete in the next Olympics. I once had a student in a YogaBellies for Pregnancy class tell me that she was planning to run a marathon three weeks' post-partum. Aside from being unsafe and being entirely unrealistic, I imagine this venture would have required a whole lot of TenaLady. Thankfully, once baby arrived, she decided to honour her body and not to run the marathon.

Even if you're not pushing yourself, you should still pay attention to signs from your body that you're not getting enough rest and that perhaps you have to slow things down a notch.

Some of these signs are the kind of thing you would expect to happen when you work out, such as a shortness of breath. There's nothing wrong with this, but it is a sign from your body that it has had to strain itself, and you should avoid going even this far, within the first few weeks after birth.

More importantly however, you should be aware of any cramps, muscle tenseness, and other 'painful' muscle related symptoms. These are more telling signs that you're moving a little too fast, and if you find yourself facing any of these symptoms while practicing asana, you should stop whatever you're doing and rest for a while. Just pop yourself into Balasana (child's pose.) Once you have rested and the cramping s gone, try another postures and see if the pain has subsided. If it has, feel free to continue, but if you persistently have the same problem, then you need to see your GP or your health visitor.

All said and done, you should basically just pay attention to your body, and how it reacts to your yoga practice. Start with gentle but firm post-natal yoga, and work back up to your arduous Ashtanga practice, if that is where you were at pre-pregnancy. Do that, and you should be just fine.

At this point, we've covered pretty much everything you need to know before you begin your post-natal yoga practice… so all that is left now is to actually start!

Bringing Movement Back into Your Life

Until you've had your first postnatal check-up, you can ease yourself into simple exercise by starting off with brisk walking. If you were very athletic previously, or in great shape, you could even consider short jogs. Take baby out in his sling or buggy and enjoy the fresh air.

Try some gentle pelvic floor exercises or 'engaging your Bandhas' (more on this soon) to start off with. Remember not to exercise bruised muscles, so if you're still sore down below, wait until there is no pain. Do these when breastfeeding or driving.

Get Your BAP's Back in Shape!

Once you are at least 6-8 weeks' post-partum after a vaginal birth or 8-10 weeks post C-section, then you can begin to practice again and tart to focus on your BAP's: Your Back, Ab's and Pelvic floor.

Post-natal yoga will ease any lower back pain; start to tone those abdominal muscles and strengthen that pelvic floor. We know how precious your time is so I put together some 10 minute YogaBellies BAP's routines that you can practice daily post-partum. I am going to show you a safer, gentler yet stronger and more effective way to strengthen those BAP's and ease any post-natal discomfort and aches and pains you may be experiencing.

I've included a simple BAP's Mother Salutation to get you started. Try practicing this simple sequence for just 10 minutes for two weeks and you will feel and see a real difference in how you look and how you feel post-natally.

What is a Mother Salutation?

Mother Salutations are practiced during YogaBellies for Mum & Baby classes. They have been careful created to gently but effectively work you're your post-natal body. These salutations are safe for pregnancy and post-partum and focus on strengthening the mind, body and especially the BAP's!

Mother Salutations honour everything that it is to be a woman and flow gracefully from one posture to the next, building in strength and stamina from one posture to the next. Perfect for the challenges you will face as a new mum.

How Do I Start to Work On My BAP's?

Get your BAP's Mother Salutation sequences to hand before you begin to practice. You only need ten minutes so this is something you can do with or without baby. You can check out the videos of the Mother Salutations on the YogaBellies YouTube channel/

I suggest that everyone start with Mother Salutation A and progress to C, as and when they feel ready. Remember you can continue this practice every day, even after 14 days, so there is no hurry to reach Mother Salutation C.

Getting back into your yoga practice post-natally is about respecting and healing your body, NOT forcing it beyond its capabilities or pushing yourself beyond what feels comfortable.

Your 14-day BAP's practice should look something like this:

Day 1-3: Mother Salutation A X 5-10 rounds
Day 4-7: Mother salutation B X 5-10 rounds
Day 8-14: Mother Salutation C X 5-10 rounds

I have stated that the practice lasts 10 minutes per day, but you can take longer if you have the time, and you will obviously benefit more from the practice. Up to 30 minutes' maximum practice time is just fine.

What the foof are 'Bandhas?'

If you've never practiced yoga before, these might be foreign terms to you. The 'bandhas' are difficult to explain in words (and they're not easy to teach either), but these two techniques are essential to start practicing postpartum! Mula bandha is essentially engaging (or lifting) your pelvic floor, and Uddiyana Bandha is essentially engaging your midsection abdominals (pulling the navel gently back and up.) Don't rush or force the bandhas, take it gently and be aware of any discomfort. If you experience any pain, stop immediately.

The bandhas are a great place to start post natally. Just spend some time trying to feel these two "locks," or bandhas. Both areas (pelvic floor and abdominals) are weakened during pregnancy and birth and by starting to engage the bandhas, we can reconnect with these areas of our body so important for our overall health, wellness and physical integrity.

When Should I Practice the Bandhas?

You can practice engaging the bandhas while reading a book, watching TV or driving—basically, at any time. When you practice your Mother Salutations, try to engage both bandhas throughout the flow. If you forget, don't panic, just re-engage them when you remember to do so :) When we engage the bandhas, we immediately stand taller and (bonus) our abs look more toned!

What are the Benefits of Bandhas?

Learning to engage the bandhas helps aid post-natal healing. This is true for women who have had a vaginal birth or a C-section. Engaging the bandhas throughout the Mother Salutations energizes and strengthens the BAP's (back, abdomen and pelvic floor,) but the great news is we can aim to become aware of the bandhas at all times!

Post-natal back pain is often caused by a combination of an over-stressed or weakened pelvic floor and abdominal muscles. This discomfort can be made worse by things like picking baby up incorrectly, changing nappies and breastfeeding in awkward positions. If we use the bandhas to become aware of our movements, we can minimize discomfort and any further damage. Hoorah! The Bandhas help you to control and improve the function of your body's internal organs and systems. We feel more balanced, digestion is regulated and our reproductive and nervous systems are re-energized.

YogaBellies Post-Natal BAP's Routines

YogaBellies Love Your BAPs

Mother Salutation A

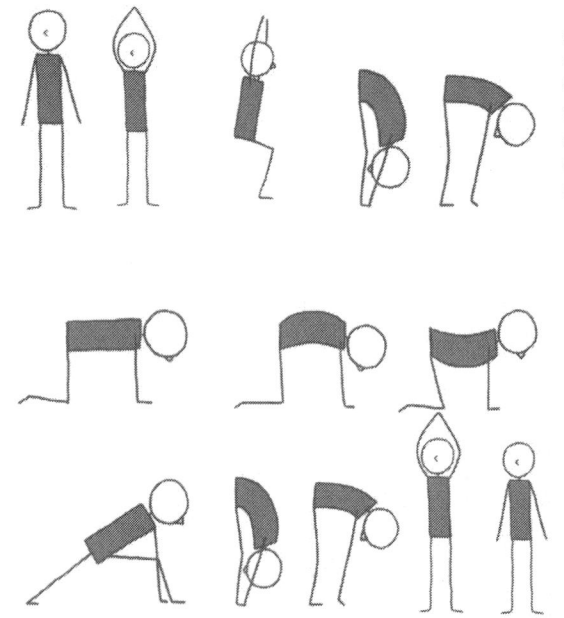

From standing pose raise the arms overhead and coming to squat, bring elbows to knees and bend forward.

Take stomach to chest in forward fold and attempt to straighten legs, hands on floor or shins/knees. Come onto fingertips and look forward.

Step back onto all fours with flat back. As we curl the spine up look towards the navel and INHALE, take navel to spine. EXHALE, take navel even further towards spine (gentle now!) INHALE and curl down, navel towards the mat and look up between the eyebrows.

Step forward into standing forward bend as before. Come onto fingertips and look forward. Bend forward one more time then raise up hands above head in prayer and back to starting position.

YogaBellies BAPs Challenge Day 1-3: Mother Salutation A

The YogaBellies Mother Salutation A is perfect for those who are less than 4 months post partum; those who are entirely new to yoga practice or have not done much physical exercise of late. You can even practice MS A if you are pregnant, (for pregnant ladies DO NOT practice the reverse breathing exercise.) It is also recommended to use Mother Salutation A for the entire challenge if you have undergone a c-section in the past 4 months or suffer from Diastis Recti (abdominal splitting.)

Mother Salutation A is a gentle yet effective way to start working every muscle group in the body with particular focus on the BAP's Back, Abs and Pelvic floor. On days 1-3 our focus is on working with the breath, becoming aware of how powerful our breath can be in effectively but safely toning the BAP's. Remember to breathe and focus on inhaling as we come UP and exhaling as we come down during the flow,. When we use REVERSE BREATHING, we do the opposite.

What do I do?

Mother Salutation A should be practised 5-10 times each day in days 1-3 of the BAP's Challenge. Easy peasy. You can stay at this level for days 1-3 or you can continue to practice A for the entire 14 day programme. The important thing is to listen to your body!

Mother Salutation B

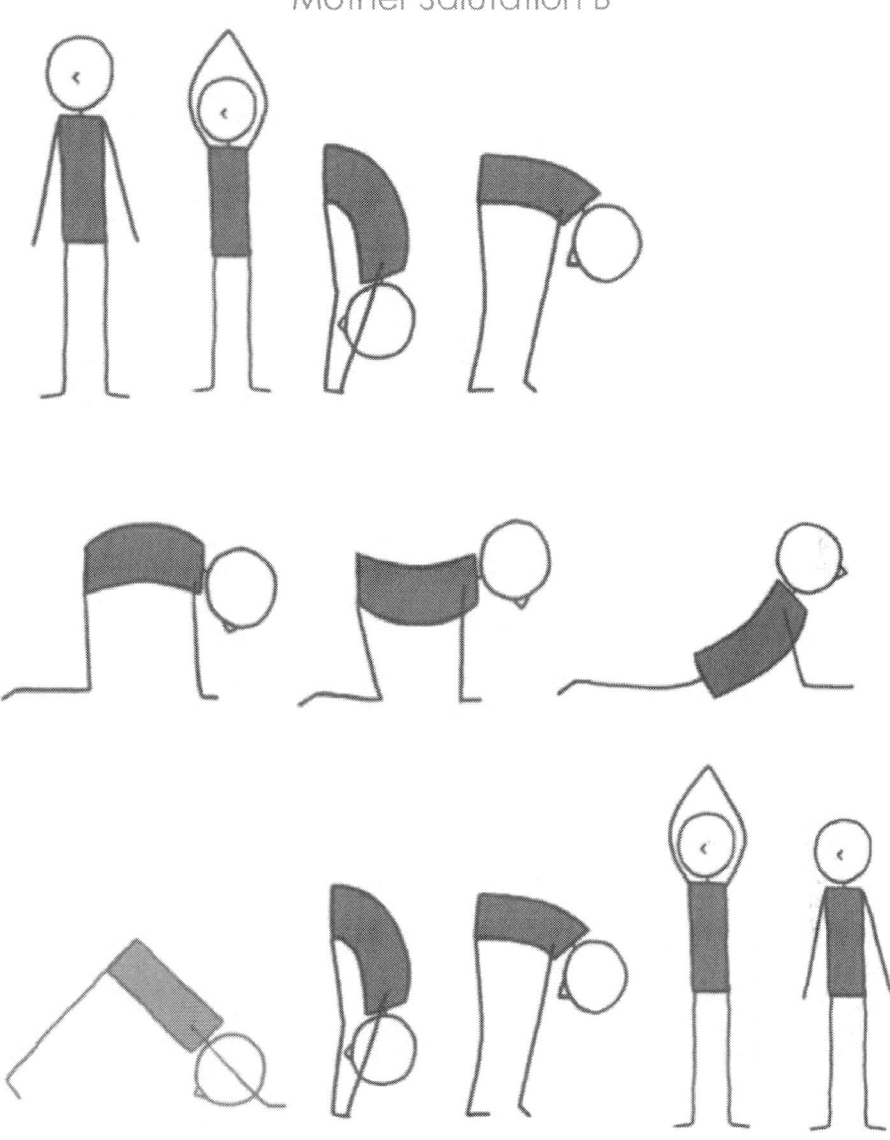

YogaBellies Love Your BAPs — Mother Salutation C

From standing pose, raise the arms overhead and bend forward, taking hands to ground. Bend knees if needed.

Take stomach to chest in forward fold and attempt to straighten legs, hands on floor or shins/knees. Come onto the fingertips and look forward.

Step back into half plank, shins on ground. Hold for 1-3 breaths and gently lower body to ground. Lie face down on mat.

Push into the hands, roll the shoulder back and gently raise head as you lift chest off the mat. Gaze forward, coming into Upward facing dog for 5 breaths.

Push into hands, pull buttocks up and back and take heels towards mat coming into Downward Dog for 5 breaths. Bend knees if you have to and don't force heels onto the mat.

From downward dog raise the right leg towards the sky, flex the foot. And come into Donkey pose Hold for 3-5 breaths. Come back to downward dog and place the feet. Do the same on the left.

Step forward into standing forward bend as before. Come onto fingertips and look forward. Bend forward one more time then raise up hands above head in prayer and back to starting position.

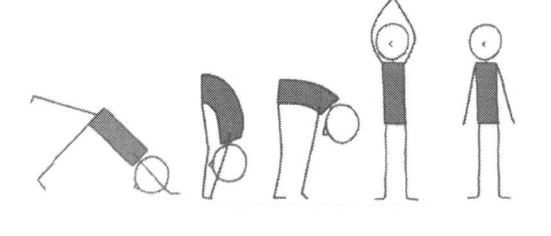

YogaBellies BAPs Challenge Day 8-14: Mother Salutation C

The YogaBellies Mother Salutation C is NOT suitable for pregnancy. It is perfect for post partum mums (more than 4 months post partum) and anyone wishing to strengthen their BAP's. Move onto Mother Salutation C when you are ready, you may be more comfortable continuing with Mother Salutation A or B for days 8-14. Proceed with caution if you suffer from Diastis Recti (abdominal splitting) and feel free to change upward dog for more cat curls or leave it out all together. If you have had a C-section please leave out half plank.

Mother Salutation C is a stronger, yet very safe way to work with the BAP's Back, Abs and Pelvic floor, adding in some stronger postures. On days 1-7, our focus has been on working with the breathe to tone the BAP's. We continue this work, but add in some strenuous downward dog and upward dog, half plank and donkey poses too, in a stronger, more dynamic practice.

What do I do?

Mother Salutation C should be practised 5-10 times each day in days 8-14 of the BAP's Challenge. You can also continue to practice REVERSE BREATHING during cat curls in addition to Mother Salutation C. You can stay at Mother Salutation A or progress to B or C as you feel comfortable. The important thing

Finding Ways to Fit Your Yoga Practice Around Your Baby

The great thing that we know about post-natal yoga, is that baby can join in, so this is not really a problem. I still fit in yoga postures while down on the floor playing Lego games with my five-year-old. Get creative and start multitasking mama!

Keep one thing in mind throughout all of this: Unless you have someone to take care of your baby, you're not going to be able to get to a yoga class yourself, which is fine. You can start to practice again at home when you have time when baby is asleep and start attending normal hatha yoga classes again after six months.

Beyond The Baby Blues

Practically every woman will experience post-partum or 'baby blues to a certain extent. Post-partum depression can last up to a year or even beyond this. Studies have shown that yoga has a hugely beneficial impact on incidence of postpartum and antenatal depression. Even if you are not suffering, one of your friends could be, so keep an eye out for the following symptoms:

The symptoms of post-partum depression include:

- Guilt
- Sadness
- Hopelessness
- Fatigue
- Emptiness
- Sleepy
- High irritability
- Impaired motor functions
- Anxiety and panic attacks
- Poor quality of sleep
- Angry or agitated
- Decreased Libido

Practicing yoga and eating well can hugely influence your susceptibility to post-natal depression. Make sure that you allow yourself to be taken care of by friend and family, don't be afraid to rely heavily on your support network and to reach out if you have to. We've all been there and just talking to someone else can be so therapeutic.

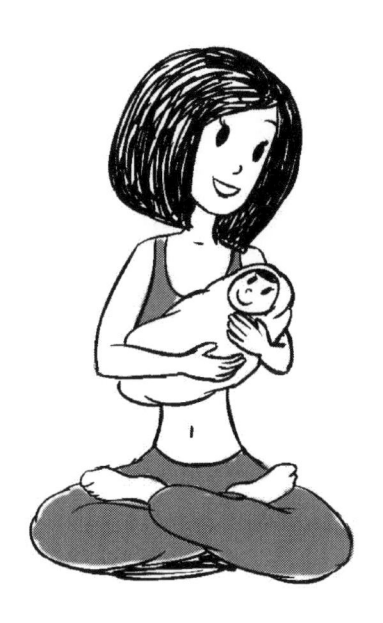

Some Final Thoughts...

Final Thoughts

Pregnancy is an amazing time in any woman's life. It is the time when you give birth to your very own little mini person: an exact replica of you both! Woohoo! From the day you find out you are pregnant, to the day you hold your child for the first time in your arms, you will enjoy and treasure every moment of your beautiful mama journey.

There will be times where you will feel like the happiest person in the world, and quite rightly so. There will also be times where you feel like screaming at everything and everyone around you. Remember that you are never alone and it's important to rely on those around you. If you don't have any other friends with babies – I was in this situation – then make sure you get out to a class, such as YogaBellies for Mum and Baby or Baby Massage, where you can meet like-minded mamas and enjoy the support of the mama community.

When you're caught up in the excitement of pregnancy, birth and new baby, don't forget that you need to focus on good nutrition throughout the pregnancy and after birth. Ensure that your diet is full of a range of fresh and healthy food. I know it will be hard to fight those cravings, but you need to stay away from unhealthy, greasy and fat-filled food.

Do not forget that daily movement is just as important as good pregnancy nutrition. Whether you go for a brisk walk in the morning or perform yoga before you go to bed, ensure that you keep your body flexible, strong and active.

By following this guide, you will have a happy and healthy pregnancy. Remember, this guide is in no way an alternative to regular check-ups and advice from your midwife or GP. It is a guide to help you decide which foods are best to eat during a pregnancy. Always consult your primary health care provider before starting any new diet.

I hope this book has been helpful to you and I wish you all the best. If you loved my book, I would like to ask you to leave me an honest review on Amazon. Feedback is so important to share our message of peace, love and YogaBellies and you can help me to do this. Have a safe and happy pregnancy!

Namaste

Cheryl xxx

Yoga Glossary

Yoga Glossary

Asana: seat; yoga posture

Ashtanga: eight-limbed yogic path;

Ayurveda: the ancient Indian science of health

Balasana: Child's pose. Take the buttocks back to the feels and place forehead on blocks or mat.

Brahmarri Breath: This breathing technique derives its name from the black Indian bee called Brahmarri. (Brahmarri = type of Indian bee; pranayama = breathing technique.) The exhalation in this pranayama resembles the typical humming sound of a bee, which explains why it is named so.

Chakra: energy centre; the basic system has seven chakras (root, sacrum, solar plexus, heart, throat, third eye and crown), each of which is associated with a colour, element, syllable, significance, etc.

Ghee: An Indian butter which promotes good digestion.

Guru: one who brings us from darkness to light; a spiritual mentor

Karma: action; the law of karma is the law of cause and effect. Karma is based upon the complex, esoteric web of conditions, individuals and relationships in the universe. It is not just as simple as a notion like "steal from someone and you'll be robbed."

Mantra: a repeated sound, syllable, word or phrase; often used in chanting and meditation.

Meditation: Focusing and calming the mind often through breath work to reach deeper levels of consciousness.

Mudra: A seal. Positions of the body that have an influence on the energies of the body, or mood. Mostly the hands and fingers are held in a mudra.

Nadi Shodana: Nadi Shodhana, or "alternate nostril breathing," is a simple but powerful technique that deeply relaxes the mind and body.

Namaste: "I bow to you"; a word used at the beginning and/or end of class which is most commonly translated as "the light within me bows to the light within you"; a common greeting in India and neighbouring cultures; a salutation said with the hands in Anjali mudra.

Om: the original syllable; chanted "A-U-M" at the beginning and/or end of many yoga classes

Padmasana (lotus pose:) This pose has become maybe the world known icon of the science and practice of yoga. As the lotus grows from the dirty waters and yet is untouched by them so should the yogi be untouched, influence or disturbed or involved by worldly things.

Practice: Refers to your 'yoga practice' or the time that you devote to practicing yoga.

Prana: life energy; chi; qi

Pranayama: breath control; breathing exercises

Rasa Dhatu: tissues or fibres that make up the physical body

Savasana: corpse pose; final relaxation; typically performed at the end of every hatha yoga class, no matter what style

Shakti: female energy

Surya Namaskara or Sun Salutations; a system of yoga exercises performed in a flow or series

Sutras: classical texts; the most famous in yoga is, of course, Patanjali's Yoga Sutras.

Ujjayi (a.k.a as Hissing Breath, Victorious Breath): A type of pranayama in which the lungs are fully expanded and the chest is puffed out; most often used in association with yoga poses, especially in the vinyasa style.

Vata: Vata governs all movement in the mind and body. It controls blood flow, elimination of wastes, breathing and the movement of thoughts across the mind. Since Pitta and Kappa cannot move without it, **Vata** is considered the leader of the three Ayurvedic Principles in the body.

Vinyasa - Vinyasa refers to a series of connected movements, performed in sequence. The sequence of warm up postures, Surya Namaskara A and B, are examples of vinyasa, as are the short sequences of movements used to connect one pose to another.

Yogi/Yogini: a male/female practitioner of yoga.

Yoga: From the Sanskrit "yug" (yoke), means "union". Yoga is an ancient discipline in which physical postures, breath practice, meditation and philosophical study are used as tools for achieving liberation.

References

References

Garabedian, Helen, Itsy Bitsy Yoga, Simon & Schuster, 2004

Yogini: The Power of Women In Yoga by Janice Gates

Magical Beginnings, Enchanted Lives: A Holistic Guide to Pregnancy and Childbirth by Deepak Chopra (Goodreads Author), David Simon

Yoga For Women by Shakta Kaur Khalsa

The Science of Yoga: The Risks and the Rewards by William J. Broad

The Heart of Yoga: Developing a Personal Practice by T.K.V. Desikachar

Larson, Jyothi, Yoga Mom, Buddha Baby: The Workout for New Mums, Bantam Books 2002

Ashtanga Yoga For Women by Sally Griffyn

The Women's Health Big Book of Yoga: The Essential Guide to Complete Mind/Body Fitness by Kathryn Budig

Yoga for Pregnancy, Birth & Beyond by Françoise Barbira Freedman

Yoga For Pregnancy by Rosalind Widdowson

Yoga Mama, Yoga Baby: Ayurveda and Yoga for a Healthy Pregnancy and Birth by Margo Shapiro Bachman

Yoga Sadhana for Mothers: Shared experiences of Ashtanga yoga, pregnancy, birth and motherhood by Sharmila Desai, Anna Wise

Yoga for Pregnancy and Birth. Uma Dinsmore-Tulli by Uma Dinsmore-Tuli

Yoga: A Gem for Women by Geeta S. Iyengar

Ram, N. Yoga Alleviates Postpartum Depression. Available online at http://www.naturalnews.com/025562_yoga_depression_postpartum_depression.html

Read, S. & Rickwood, D. Participation in Community-Based Parenting Groups as Protective Factor for Women's Postnatal Mental Health. In Women and Depression. Iffat Hussain (Ed.). Cambridge Scholars Publishing; UK, 2010.

Sharp, A. Postnatal Depression. In T. Kendrick, A. Tylee, & P. Freeling (Eds.). The
Prevention of Mental Illness in Primary Care. New York: Cambridge University Press, 1996.

Streeter et al. Effects of Yoga Versus Walking on Mood, Anxiety, and Brain GABA Levels: A Randomized Controlled MRS Study. The Journal of Alternative and Complementary Medicine, 16(11): 1145-1152, 2010.

YogaBellies Birth Outcomes Survey (2012): Survey conducted over 400 mothers collating results of effects of perinatal yoga on birth outcomes and baby development.

http://www.nutraingredients-usa.com/news/ng.asp?id=60554
http://www.nutraingredients-usa.com/news/ng.asp?id=25810
http://www.nutraingredients-usa.com/news/ng.asp?id=20934
http://www.elephantjournal.com/2013/12/a-glossary-of-34-frequently-used-yoga-terms/
https://www.ayurvedacollege.com

More from

YogaBellies

About the Author

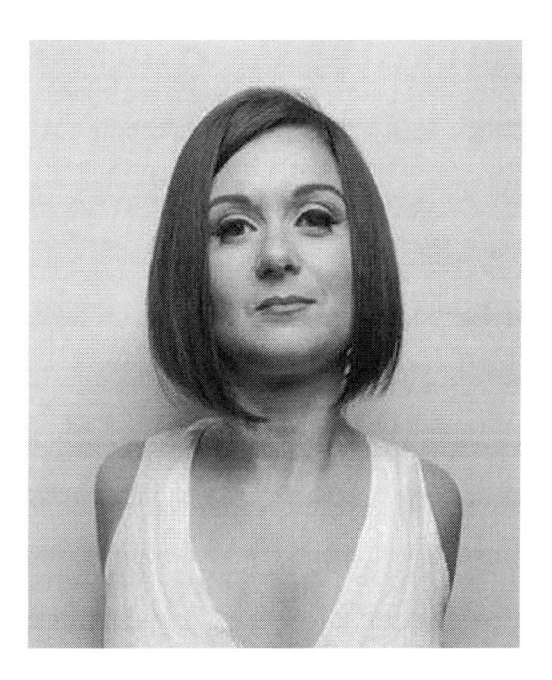

Cheryl MacDonald is a Yoga Elder, an author, a successful and ethical business woman (take a peek at Cheryl on BBC"s Dragons" Den or on ITV's 'This Morning' with Holly Willoughby.) She has been practising yoga for 18 years and has trained extensively in yoga and antenatal education amongst other holistic therapies. Her skills and experience combined with her love of yoga and the belief that everyone can practice yoga, are the essence of YogaBellies®. Cheryl has worked with celebrities such as Kimberley Walsh (of Girls Aloud fame), Fearne Cotton and Catherine Tyldsley (Coronation Street) in birth preparation and on their yoga practice too.

Cheryl is an ethical 'mumpreneur' and has been awarded multiple awards and accreditation's including The Scottish Edge Award, three

What's on 4 Little One's Awards as well as being finalist in Woman of the Year, Working Mum's Best Employer and What's on 4 Junior's Awards.

Cheryl started YogaBellies® for women who wanted to practice and experience the many benefits of yoga, without it seeming too 'mystical' or unattainable whilst also wholly embracing the feminine. She started to teach classes specifically for women, mums' and their children, so that they could grow to love yoga, connect with their true selves and to bond with each other. Cheryl has also gone on to create the Birth ROCKS Academy (affectionately known as BRA,) and PeaceLoveYoga Retreats, where she runs yoga retreats for women in Bali and Thailand.

Cheryl created the YogaBellies and YogaBelles style of yoga around the fluidity and flexibility of the female body and soul and also around the key life stages of a woman. YogaBellies® has grown to include a training faculty of teachers with a wealth of experience, including yoga teachers, doctors, midwives, massage therapists and chiropractors.

Cheryl on Yoga for Women...

"I love teaching women yoga. YogaBellies is so much more than just a yoga class, we stretch ourselves – body, mind and soul – but the most important aspect, is women supporting women. Women undergo key challenges in life: menstruation, pregnancy, being a new mother and menopause.

These times can be emotional and physically demanding times with huge adjustments. Women have become disjointed in their acknowledgement and acceptance of these stages, and the whole concept of YogaBellies is to allow ourselves to embrace and enjoy each new stage as it comes. To love being a woman and to enjoy the friendships and support of other women."

Other Books by the Author

Birth ROCKS *Paperback (2013)*
by **Cheryl Kennedy MacDonald**   (Author)
    ***** 40 customer reviews

The NEW 2015 Revised edition includes bonus chapters and a foreword by Doula and Birth Keeper, Nicola Goodall.

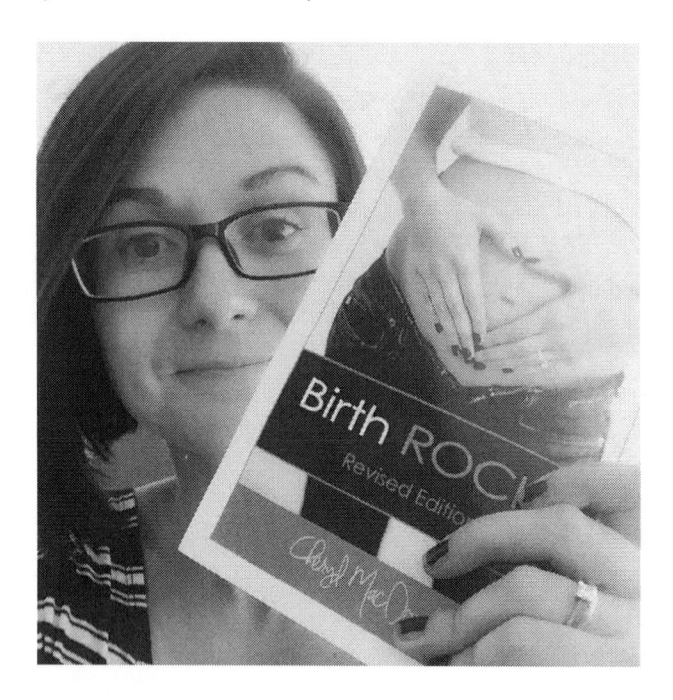

Birth ROCKS© is the revolutionary childbirth preparation method that's been taking the world by storm. Created by YogaBellies founder Cheryl MacDonald, Birth ROCKS© is an approach to childbirth that's positive, honest and most importantly, unique to you. This best-selling book accompanies your personal journey though pregnancy and birth.

The Birth ROCKS© Method helps you to understand your personal coping style in new or stressful situations; how to actively involve your partner in your birth and how to identify and release your fears of birthing.

Birth ROCKS© will help you to:

• Look forward to childbirth with excitement and feel prepared for The Big Day;

• Learn from positive birth stories from other women, reinforcing the fact that birth can be most amazing experience of your life;

• Find out if hypnobirthing is the right comfort technique for you in birth and if not, then what your other options are;

• Allow you to birth comfortably and with minimal discomfort;

• Feel confident and positive about your choices during birth;

• Encourage your pregnancy and birth to progress smoothly and naturally

To find out more about Birth ROCKS© or to find your nearest Birth ROCKS© mentor, please visit www.birthrocks.com. The Birth ROCKS book is available in Paperback and Kindle from Amazon or from Cheryl's website www.peaceloveyogaguru.com

YogaBellies for Pregnancy DVD

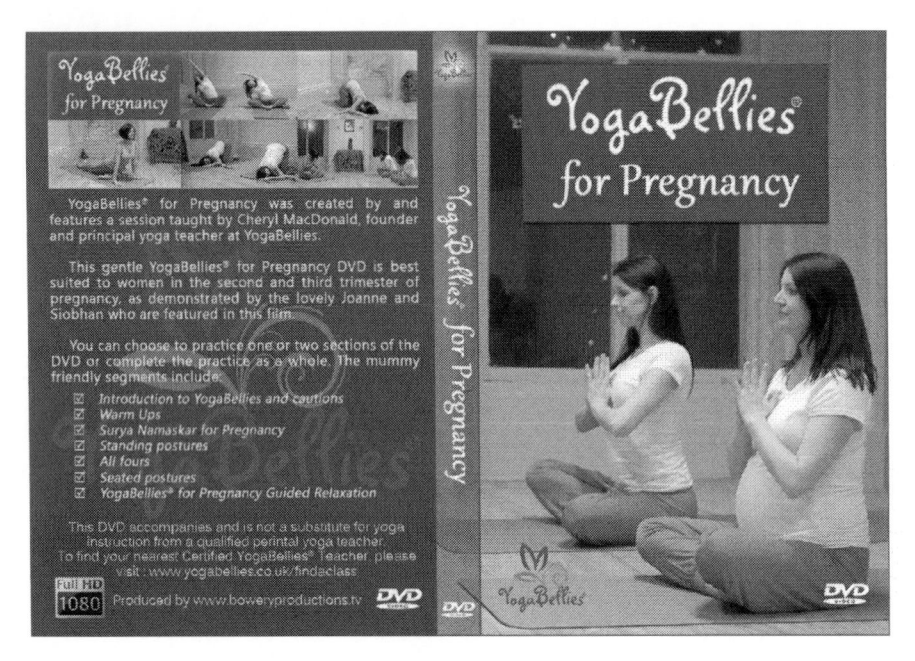

If you can't find a Certified YogaBelies Teacher nearby, then I have a DVD which you can use to accompany your pregnancy yoga practice at home.

Cheryl MacDonald, founder of YogaBellies and Yoga Elder, takes you through a beautiful pregnancy yoga practice with a difference... Along with her beautiful friends Siobhan (16 weeks pregnant) and Joanne (32 weeks pregnant), the girls take you on a peaceful journey of yoga and love at the most important time of your life.

Download now for from the YogaBellies website or buy the DVD for on Amazon.

If you'd like to download a free YogaBellies for Pregnancy mini video routine, just
pop your email address in here

Namaste

Printed in Poland
by Amazon Fulfillment
Poland Sp. z o.o., Wrocław